History of
RUSSIAN COSTUME

History of
RUSSIAN COSTUME
from the Eleventh to the Twentieth Century

From the collections of the

ARSENAL MUSEUM, LENINGRAD

HERMITAGE, LENINGRAD

HISTORICAL MUSEUM, MOSCOW

KREMLIN MUSEUMS, MOSCOW

PAVLOVSK MUSEUM

The Metropolitan Museum of Art

LIBRARY OF CONGRESS CATALOGING IN PUBLICATION DATA

Main entry under title:

History of Russian costume from the eleventh to the twentieth century.

   1. Costume—Russia—Exhibitions. I. Aleshina, T. S. II. New York (City). Metropolitan Museum of Art.

GT1040.H57 391'.00947'07401471 76-58330
ISBN 0-87099-160-4

© the Ministry of Culture of the U.S.S.R.

Designed by Peter Oldenburg

Composition by Custom Composition Company

Printed by Nicholas/David Lithographers

Catalogue compiled by

T.S. ALYOSHINA,
scientific worker of the Historical Museum, Section of Urban Costume

I.I. VISHNEVSKAYA,
scientific worker of the Kremlin Museums, Section of Old Russian Costume

L.V. EFIMOVA,
scientific worker of the Historical Museum, Section of Old Russian Costume

T.T. KORSHUNOVA,
scientific worker of the Hermitage, Section of Urban Costume

V.A. MALM,
scientific worker of the Historical Museum, Section of Archaeology

E.Yu. MOISEENKO,
scientific worker of the Hermitage, Section of National Dress

M.M. POSTNOKOVA-LOSEVA,
scientific worker of the Historical Museum, Section of Jewelry

E.P. CHERNUKHA,
scientific worker of the Kremlin Museums, Section of Old Russian Costume

Cover: Catherine the Great's full-dress uniform of the Equestrian Regiment of the Life Guards (299)

All photographs, except for those by Malcolm Varon, which are on pages 17, 18, 35, 36, 85, 88 right, 89, and cover, are courtesy of the State Hermitage Museum, Leningrad, and the State Historical Museum, Moscow.

INTRODUCTION

The *Glory of Russian Costume* exhibition is created on the basis of materials from the collections of leading museums of the USSR: the Pavlovsk Museum, the Arsenal Museum, Leningrad, the State Museums of the Moscow Kremlin, the State Historical Museum, Moscow, and the State Hermitage, Leningrad. Its exhibits are a small part of the collections of these museums, which include all periods of the development of world culture.

The sources of Russian folk art go back deep into the past centuries of the culture of Slavic tribes. Popular domestic peasant art was born from the way of life of the people itself, in the process of work based on a natural striving toward beauty and creativity. This determined the peculiarity of the contents and of the artistic language of this art. Beautiful everyday objects reflected the spiritual culture and the aesthetic ideals of both the peasants and of the village and town craftsmen.

The influence of folk art and the artistic culture of Russia is strongly evident in the 17th century. Masters coming from among the people built and decorated magnificent architectural ensembles, churches, tsars' palaces, mansions of the boyars, and created and decorated objects for use in their daily lives. For the needs of the nobility unique textiles and embroideries, ornamental jewelry, and items of clothing were made. The high level of folk, or peasant, art served as a stimulus for the creation of craft centers that were the basis for development during the 18th and 19th centuries of manufacturing centers and many branches of Russian artistic industry.

Costume, as an artistic phenomenon, is obviously related to the general direction of the development of Russian decorative art. As part of the material culture of the society, it reflects the history of the people.

In this connection, the exhibition presented to the American audience goes far beyond the framework of a narrowly professional one, and is definitely of great interest to the widest circles of the population. The exhibition acquaints the visitor with the traditional shapes of Russian clothing, as well as with the character of the later all-European type of costume in Russia.

The collection includes more than 500 authentic examples of clothing dating from the 11th to the beginning of the 20th century from the collections of the leading museums of the USSR.

The basic part of the collection consists of real masterpieces of folk art that are of great artistic value and bear witness to the great multifaceted artistic talents of the Russian people.

Among the exhibits are ensembles and individual items of clothing, details of decorative patterns on textiles, precious embroideries, headdresses, and shoes. The history of Russian costume of the early period is represented by items from archaeological excavations. Another part of the exhibition consists of unique monuments of Russian history carefully preserved in the museums' collections. The visitor to the exhibition will become acquainted with the clothes of Peter I (Peter the Great) and will see the wedding gown of Catherine II, the military uniform of the great Russian general Suvorov, and other exhibits connected with historically prominent persons.

This exhibition of Russian costume is being shown abroad for the first time, but in our country the articles contained in it, as well as an enormous number of other items of clothing and of decorative arts, are gathered in our museums and are well known to a wide circle of museum visitors. These objects serve as authentic sources of inspiration as well as basic material for the creativity not only for artists who design contemporary costume, textiles, and jewelry, but also for artists working for the theater and for the movies, and painters and sculptors who re-create in their works people and events of our country's history. The teams of dancers that are known worldwide, such as that of I. Moiseyev or the "Berezka" (Little Birch Tree), as well as many popular choral groups and individual performers, are dressed in costumes executed according to popular traditions.

Costume is of an enormous importance for the re-creation of national flavor and for the creation of historical background for such well-known operas by Russian composers as: "Boris Godunov," "Khovanshchina," and "Pskovityanka" (The Woman of Pskov), as well as for such fairy-tale operas as "Ruslan and Ludmila," "The Snow Maiden," "Sadko," etc. National costumes are used in many theatrical performances and movies.

This exhibition does not attempt to give a complete picture of the history of the development of Russian popular and urban costume, but attempts to acquaint the visitor with basic stages of its development. The exhibits included in it, serve, in a way, as bright stakes denoting the most characteristic periods of such history.

The art of Russian costume is arranged chronologically in three sections:
Russian Costume from the 11th to the 17th Century
Folk Costume from the 18th to the Early 20th Century
Urban Costume from the 18th to the Early 20th Century

Russian Costume from the 11th to the 17th Century

One can judge the character of the clothing of Slavic tribes of the 11th-13th century by the archaeological material from this period. No costume exists preserved in its entirety, but there is a representation of a dressed man and there are details and fragments that permit us to reconstruct the sources of decorative principles and of the ornamental forms in the Russian costume.

Fragments of textiles demonstrate the popularity of patterned woven textiles and embroideries as early as in the 11th-13th century, with patterns in which one encounters geometric and vegetative shapes. The embroidery made with gold and silver thread found wide diffusion subsequently, and its use was preserved in the Russian dress up to the 19th century. A large collection of Slavic ornamental items executed in gold and in silver is in this exhibition. Among these are massive hoop-shaped torques, pendant rings worn on the temple, bracelets, and finger rings. Ornamental objects of one kind or another were characteristic of the dress of various tribes. The Vyatichi (a Slavic tribe) for instance used to wear temple rings with seven segments, while they complemented their dress made of white linen with strings of beads made of red carnelian or of rock crystal. Women of other tribes preferred beads of gilt or bright blue glass. One of the early representations of ancient Russian woman's costume can be seen on a bracelet made of wide silver plaques with incised ornamental design (12th or early 13th century). The design placed within arches includes representations of birds, animals, and human figures. Of interest is the figure of a dancing woman wearing a long shirt tied with belt and having very long wide sleeves; over the sleeve is worn an arm bracelet. Despite the conventionality of the design, one is able to form an idea of the general character of the costume, and a long sleeve is clearly visible. This is a very important detail, because long sleeves, reaching almost down to the floor, are characteristic of women's and men's clothing in ancient Russia and later.

Russian costume of a later period—of the 16th-17th century—is represented in the exhibition by unique examples of civilian clothing and ecclesiastical vestments. A boy's shirt made of white linen (17th century) is cut in a way typical for men's clothing, a way almost unchanged for several centuries.

The shirt was cut in straight lengths of cloth, with triangular side gussets, and with, in the armhole under the sleeve, a square gusset made of red tabby-weave fabric, set in to secure freedom of movement; in the upper part of the back and of the front are double layers of fabric, called *podopleka* (shoulder lining). Characteristic is the traditional decoration: along the seams is edging made of red tabby-weave fabric, and gold braid is applied on the shoulders. The shirt was worn with the hem hanging loose over the trousers, and with a belt placed low. To the set of men's clothing belonged also a caftan.

In the exhibition is a seafarer's caftan, found on the Taimyr peninsula at the site of a temporary station of the explorer's expedition of the 17th century. It is made of rough homespun woolen cloth and could have belonged not only to a seafaring man, but also to a plowman.

A striking example of ancient Russian dress is provided by a woman's silk *okhaben,* or summer cloak (17th century). This item is made for outer wear: the cloak is long, open in front, wide at the bottom, with long sleeves. It is cut on straight lines of straight lengths of cloth, with triangular side inserts and side slits; the borders are trimmed with gold galloon. A man's coat could have been cut in an identical manner, a similarity noted by contemporaries. A common pattern was characteristic in Russia for the dress of various social groups as well; the only exception was the courtiers' costume.

Outstanding in its originality is the field caftan of Tsar Peter I (of about 1689) from the collection of the Armory of the Moscow Kremlin. It is long, open in front, cut on straight lines, with wedge-shaped side inserts, very wide short sleeves, and a fitted back. It is decorated with bobbin lace made of metallic gold thread. Of great interest is the cloth of which the caftan is sewn. The *bois de rose*-colored silk, known as *baiberek,* was woven in Moscow by Russian masters. This constitutes a rare case for the 17th century, because the silk-weaving industry was developed only in the 18th century. The textile of which the caftan is made is one of the few existing examples of the first steps taken by the Moscow court in the last quarter of the 17th century on its road to creating a native industry.

In the exhibition are represented examples of ecclesiastical vestments of the 17th century, and among them the costume of Patriarch Nikon (mid-17th century). It is made of dark blue velvet and is noteworthy for its original cut.

The tsar's attire and the clothes of the boyars and of the church notables were distinguished by the luxury of imported brocades, silks, and velvets. Russian merchants imported these at different times in great quantities from Byzantium, Iran, Turkey, Italy, and other countries with which Russia kept up widespread commercial and political relations. However, among pieces in this section attention is attracted by items executed by Russian male and female artisans: magnificent examples of metallic gold embroidery, fragments of Russian block printed linen, and ornamental pieces, among which stand out by their originality silver buttons and earrings. Individual costume details fill in the idea of how the woman's costume looked: the headdress of Tsarina Anastasiya Romanovna (1560) made of braided silk and gold threads, the woman's boot made of red velvet and embroidered with pearls, knitted silk gloves trimmed with lace, and many other items, bear witness of the rich artistic inheritance of the Russian people.

Folk Costume from the 18th to the Early 20th Century

The abundance of surviving examples of folk art of this period permits us to form a most complete idea of that time, as compared to the preceding epochs. The character of folk art of the 17th century was formed in complicated ways; the gap was widening between the folk culture and that of the nobility, but at the same time the two remained in a complicated interpenetration. Nevertheless, a certain conservatism of the peasants' way of life caused a stability in the basic forms of clothing, and of the folkloristic character of ornamentation.

In the exhibition is the traditional national peasants' costume in all its many-faceted variety. Here are displayed for the most part women's holiday clothes in which one can see expressed to a high degree the people's astounding optimism, joy of living, and inborn taste and sensitivity. Despite the general similarity in the manner of cut and in the decoration, the costumes from various regions of Russia differ considerably in character, colors, and details. Most important are the differences found between the clothing of the northern and southern districts, while in Central Russia one can observe aspects close to both types.

The peasant women of the Russian North—of the Arkhangelsk, Vologda, Novgorod, and Tver districts—wore a costume that consisted of a shirt, a *sarafan*, an apron, and a belt.

The shirts were made of linen and were generously embroidered in colored linen, silk, and gold thread and with galloons and spangles. The patterns of the embroideries vary. Usually ornamental strips were applied at the collar and at the border of the sleeve. Special attention was given to the trimming of the hem: multifigured compositions include representations of birds, horses, fantastic trees, and solemn female figures with their arms raised and invariably accompanied by horsemen. In these subjects are reflected the beliefs of the pagan Slavs concerning the forces of nature and the fertility of earth brought about by the sun in the spring: conceptions that were related to agricultural labors of the Slavic plowman.

Shirts were also made of patterned linen, muslin, and silk. Long sleeves reaching down beyond the palm of the hand are a tribute to the ancient Russian tradition.

The young girls came out for the mowing or for the first letting out to the pasture of the cattle wearing festive long shirts tied with a belt. On other occasions, the shirt was worn with a *sarafan*.

The *sarafan* is connected with the image of the Russian

costume. The most festive *sarafan*s of the 18th century were made of silk fabrics manufactured in Russian factories. They were cut wider toward the hem (cut on bias at the sides, or gored), opening in front, with ornamental closures. The patterns on the fabrics were enhanced with precious buttons, laces, and galloons. Such *sarafan*s were worn on holidays by wealthy peasant women and city dwellers of the lower middle class. These costumes were carefully preserved, and were left as inheritance from one generation to another.

In the exhibition are some *sarafan*s no less valuable from an artistic point of view, even if they are of a more modest variety, made of crude linen with block printing (made by hand) in a vegetative pattern. To the basic costume of peasant women of the Russian North—the shirt and the *sarafan*—were added in many localities richly embroidered aprons.

On important holidays, over the *sarafan* was worn a *dushegreya* (warm jacket). These short jackets with long sleeves were usually made of scarlet silk damask or red velvet. The color red used in the costumes of Russian peasants from time immemorial symbolized goodness and beauty.

On the whole, the North Russian costume is distinguished by its reserved colors and graceful silhouette. In its structure and image is found a reflection of the soft and somewhat severe beauty of the Northern Russian nature. A totally different emotional image is contained in the costume of the peasants of the central and the southern districts of Russia: those of Ryazan, Kaluga, Kursk, and Voronezh.

To the set of South Russian costume besides the shirt, belonged the *poneva*, a kind of a skirt, made up of three lengths of checked woolen homespun sewn together. This is one of the most archaic parts of clothing of eastern Slavs. The peasant women usually owned several *poneva*s which they wore on strictly defined special occasions: on holidays, a dressier one, with bright decoration of multicolored embroidery and woven strips, and on weekdays, one that was modestly trimmed in *kumach* (red fustian). Over the shirt and the *poneva* was worn a closed apron with a top, the decorative patterns of which were remarkable by their varied and bright colors. The figure of the woman wearing such a costume acquired a solemn and monumental aspect. In the exhibition are represented several costumes from Southern and Central Russia consisting of complete sets: a shirt, a *poneva,* an apron, and outer clothing.

Local originality is reflected in the costume of the Voronezh district. Here the woman's shirt is decorated with embroidery executed in black thread and can be distinguished by its reserve and refinement.

Among the exhibits one finds an exceptionally rich collection of women's headdresses. The headdress is one of the most traditional details of a Russian costume. Each region had a particular shape for it, and everywhere the headdress worn by maidens was considerably different from the one worn by married women. The reason for this was the ancient custom, common to all eastern Slavic peoples, according to which a married woman was obliged to hide her hair from the eyes of a stranger; one could not enter a house or attend to household duties with one's head uncovered. The maidens plaited their hair into a single braid and could keep their heads uncovered. From this custom the shape of the headdress was derived: for a married woman, a kind of small closed cap and for a young girl, a light band or hoop that leaves the top of the head uncovered. The changes in hair arrangement and in the headdress were part of the wedding ritual and were always accompanied by special rites and lamentations.

One of the types of headdress that was widely popular was the *kokoshnik.* In northern regions it was embroidered all over with pearls, which were obtained from the northern rivers, and with metallic gold thread, while a net woven from strings of pearls came down low over the forehead. The *kokoshnik*s of the central regions were tall, while those in the Vladimir and Nizhny Novgorod districts had a rounded, crescent-shaped outline, and those of Kostroma were peaked. They too were decorated with pearls, semiprecious stones, bits of mirror, and multicolored foil or tinsel; the back was made of silk or of velvet richly embroidered in gold thread. The *kokoshnik* was the most precious part of the clothing and in it continued to survive the ancient gold and pearl embroidery techniques. Pearl-embroidered *kokoshnik*s were worn mainly by wealthy middle-class women and merchants' wives living in towns, while in the villages they were worn on special holidays and at weddings. In portraits painted by Russian artists, exhibited in the show, dresses of the 19th century are shown with the costume. A bride's *kokoshnik* on one of the portraits is covered by a light muslin veil with allover embroidery.

In the south of Russia *kokoshnik*s were also worn, but their structures were more complicated; in each region they had their own individual shape and original decoration. Amazing because of their fantastic shape are those of Ryazan and Tambov, the so-called *soroki* (magpies) with horns and long "tails" made of red fustian ribbons. Less characteristic are those from Voronezh and Kursk made of gold galloon and decorated with multicolored strips. Of varied appearances, but simpler in shape, are headdresses for maidens. Among these is a northern *koruna* (crown) embroidered in pearls, and also embroidered braid covers.

In the exhibition are representative examples of necklaces, chains, and other breast ornaments made of pearls, mother-of-pearl plaquettes, glass beads, and amber.

Compared to the women's clothing that of the men looks monotonous. The *kosovorotka* shirt (with neck closing placed assymetrically, to one side), was worn everywhere, made both of homewoven and bought cotton, silk, or wool. It is noteworthy that the tuniclike cut of the shirts of this period in its details is exactly the same as that of the ancient Russian man's shirt. In the second half of the 19th century the most fashionable shirt in Russia was that made of crimson cashmere with black embroideries on its front and sleeves. Shirts

Peter the Great's dressing gown (292)
and court costume (282, 283, 284)

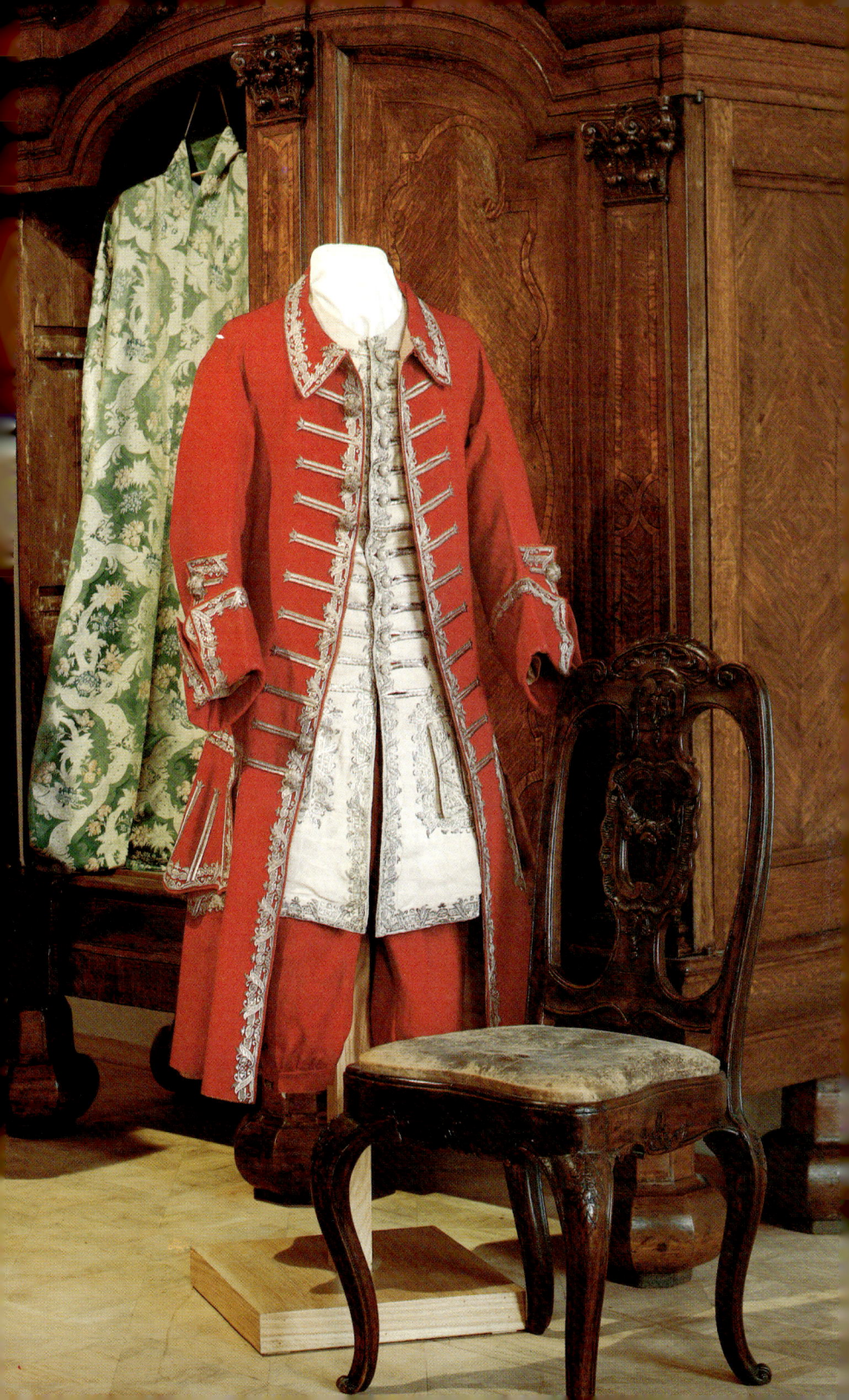

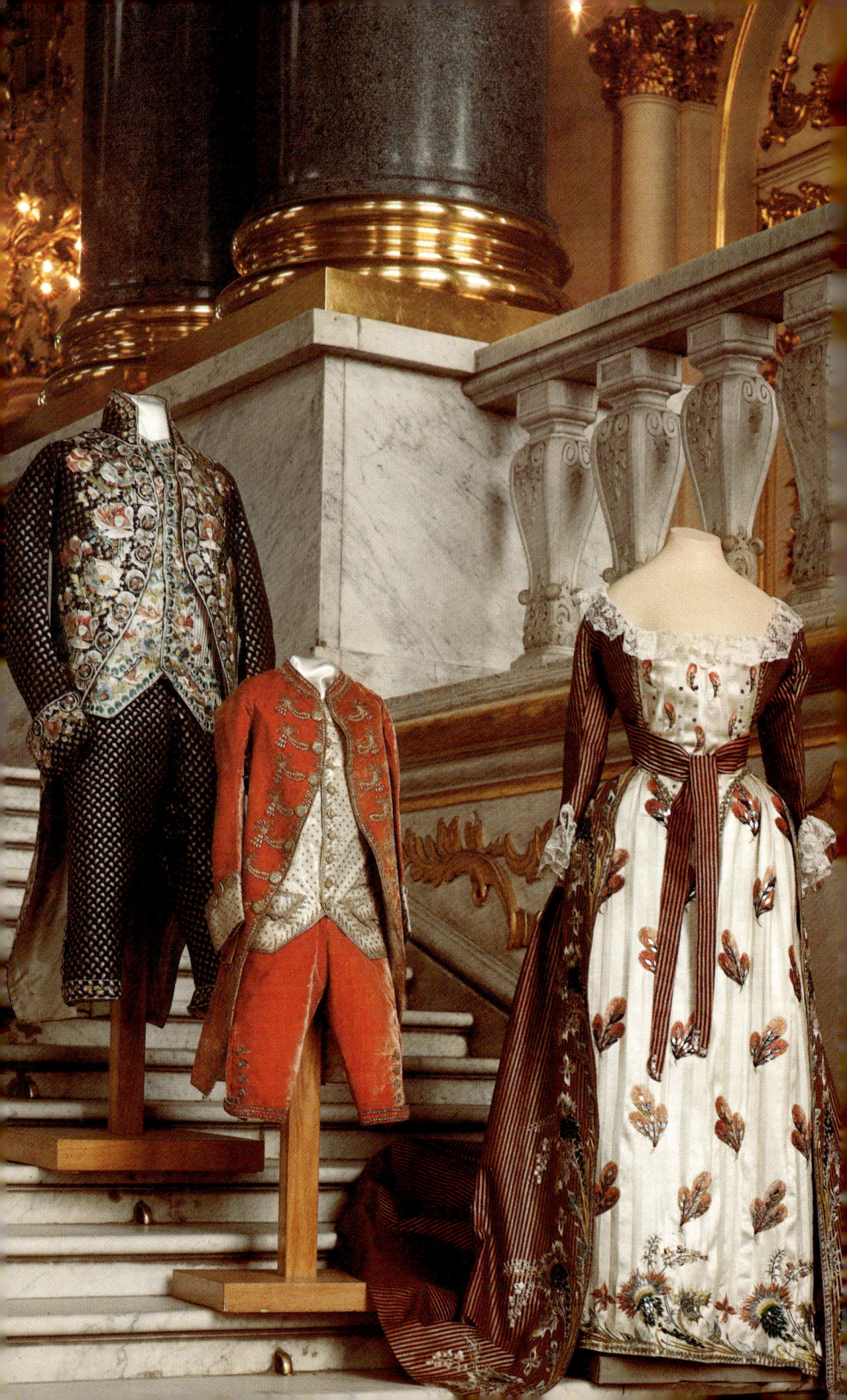

were worn with their hems loose over the trousers, and the various belts worn with these shirts could be either narrow or wide.

Up to the end of the 19th and the beginning of the 20th century in the traditional national (peasant) costume were preserved traits of ancient Russian dress, which are evident in the straight cut, the long sleeves, the manner of wearing several pieces of clothing simultaneously, and the series of chest decorations. Nevertheless, under the influence of a number of factors, the people's clothing underwent changes.

The development of industries in factories and of the urban fashion strongly influenced the peasants' way of life. This is reflected in the manufacture of textiles and of clothing: the cotton fabric production competed with that of linen and hemp; homespun linen was replaced by brightly colored chintzes and other factory-produced textiles. Under the influence of the urban fashion of the 1880s and 90s, there was born and became widespread in the villages the so-called *parochka* ("a pair") suit consisting of a skirt and blouse made of the same fabric. The woman's shirt also underwent changes: a new type of cut appeared, with a yoke; the top part of the shirt was made of calico or red fustian. The traditional complicated headdresses gradually were eliminated in favor of the cotton and woolen block printed kerchiefs that were simpler to wear. The peasant women gladly bought kerchiefs made of fustian with colorful flower patterns. Men's clothing that had preserved for a long time the traces of ancient traditions was subjected during this period to great changes; the peasant men wore jackets (*pidjak*) and visored caps.

In the exhibition one may become acquainted with the women's costume of the new type—the *parochka*—or one with the *kazachok*, consisting of a skirt and a blouse made of bright

Left: Man's court costume (309, 310, 311).
Center: Boy's court costume (312, 313, 314).
Right: Woman's court dress (306)

silk material, or a colorful shirt *pokosnitsa* (worn at mowing time) with a red fustian top and a bodice made of *pestryad* (cotton fabric with woven factory-made varicolored woolen threads), and with kerchiefs made of fustian block printed by hand and trimmed by the peasant women themselves with fringes and tassels made of dyed wool. Russian kerchiefs became widely known, especially the woolen kerchieves decorated with block printed roses, whose manufacture started in the 19th century in the small suburban town of Pavlov Posad. The famous Pavlov kerchiefs and shawls, which are still being manufactured, have won prizes at international exhibitions.

The changes in the clothing at the end of the 19th and the beginning of the 20th century are most characteristic for central industrial regions. In the south, where the peasants of the fertile "black-earth" region were devoted to agriculture, the way of life was more secluded and the urban influence not so strong, and the traditional forms of clothing were preserved until 1917.

Urban Costume from the 18th to the Early 20th Century

The evolution in the peasants' costume in Russia and its approximation to the urban one was a lengthy process, resulting from a series of independent factors.

This section begins with the earliest costumes of "Western" type, introduced in Russia by the ukases of Peter I in order to replace the traditional cumbersome boyars' dress. Beginning in 1700, several ukases were issued, strict adherence to them was carefully supervised, and those guilty of breaking them were fined.

Men's costume introduced by the reforms of Peter I, originated in its general lines at the court of Louis XIV at the end of the 17th century and consisted of a coat (caftan), a waistcoat (*kamzol*), and pants. The coat was knee-length, narrow at the waistline, with groups of deep pleats on the front skirt flaps. Tall cuffs and fancifully shaped flaps over the pockets were fastened by buttons. The *kamzol* was cut shorter than the coat, without pleats or collar, and with long narrow sleeves. The pants were worn short, just below the knee. In the exhibition are shown the everyday and the gala costumes that belonged to Peter I.

Common townspeople wore costumes made of broadcloth and linen and decorated them with buttons and sometimes with fabrics of a contrasting color. The clothing of the distinguished townspeople used more expensive fabrics: silk, velvet, and brocade. Gold and silver laces and all kinds of embroidery were used as decoration.

Military dress was also strictly regulated by Peter's ukases; in its cut it was similar to the civilian costume, but was made of wool in the specific color assigned to one or another army branches.

The reform touched on the costume of women as well. To replace the *dushegreya* (padded jacket) and the *sarafan* were introduced splendid French gowns, with bodices tightly laced at the waistline, low decolletages, sleeves to the elbow, and wide skirts. These dresses, like the men's costumes, were often decorated with cleverly executed embroidery and lace.

In the beginning, the edicts concerning the clothing aroused displeasure, but already toward the end of Peter I's reign they firmly established themselves in the daily life not only of the nobility, functionaries, and military, but also of the progressive merchants and industrialists. Beginning with the time of Peter I, the urban costume developed in Russia in the same direction as in Europe.

Both women's and the men's fashion were rather stable in the 18th century; the established type of clothing existed, with but insignificant changes, up to the 1780s. The men's costume of this period was notable by being very colorful and was often made of the same textiles as that of the women—brocade, velvet, and silk—and was richly decorated with embroidery in colored silk, gold and silver thread, spangles, and mirrors. Many Russian nobles had workshops on their estates, where the embroideries were executed by master craftsmen from among the women serfs, who sometimes introduced in the ornamental design elements of traditional Russian embroidery.

In the women's costume of this period the open gown type with a wide silk skirt predominates, which for the winter was made with cotton quilting. In order to provide the skirt with the shape fashionable in the 1730s—widening at the sides—one used paniers and farthingales: special contrivances made of willow twigs, whalebone, and firm fabric. The wide sweep of the farthingale reached one and a half meters. One of the characteristic details of the European costume of those years—the "Watteau" fold—also decorated women's gowns in Russia for several decades. The fanciful silhouette and the character of ornamentation of the fabrics and of the decoration of the costumes harmonized with the furniture and the interior decoration in the rococo style.

During this period, Catherine II attempted to introduce at the court the so-called Russian dress, a fact proven not only by the edicts of those years, but also by the so-called "dress uniform" dresses of the empress that have been preserved to our day. These were made of fabrics of the same color as the dress uniforms of individual regiments and were decorated with regulation galloons and buttons. In this peculiar costume were combined fancifully the shapes of the dominant French fashion (open dress mounted on farthingales) with elements peculiar to ancient Russian costume, such as sleeves that could be thrown back behind the shoulders, and the arrangement of the decoration.

At the end of the 1770s and the beginning of the 1780s an appreciable influence on clothing was exerted both by the ideas of J.-J. Rousseau that had spread in Russia and by the increased English influence. Especially noticeable were the new tendencies that spread after the French bourgeois revolution of 1789. In the costumes of this time a new style was strongly reflected—that of classicism. In its striving for simplicity fashion turned its attention to the aesthetic rules of antiquity.

The resplendent gowns were replaced by tunic-shaped ones. Instead of heavy silks, velvets, and brocades, appeared thin, airy linens and cottons, white for the most part, corresponding more fully to the new character of the costume. Farthingales, corsets, and whalebones in the bodices disappear. Dresses with waistlines raised high, low decolletages, and short sleeves became fashionable. The skirt fell from under the waistline in soft fluid folds and ended in a train. The costume of this type quickly spread across Europe and, despite the opposition of Paul I, who was frightened by the events of the revolution and forbade everything that was French, this fashion did not by-pass Russia either. The characteristic traits of this fashion have found a striking incorporation in the dress of embroidered white tulle made at the end of the 18th or the beginning of the 19th century, which, according to tradition, belonged to the daughter of A. V. Suvorov.

Beginning with the end of the 18th and up to the middle of the 19th century an indispensable part of women's festive gowns in Russia were woolen scarves and shawls. These were worn both in summer and in winter, and one did not part from them during balls, either. In the beginning these were imported Oriental shawls, but later ones were produced in Europe and Russia. Especially valued were Russian shawls made by female artisans from among the serfs of the landed ladies: Merlina, Eliseyeva, and Kolokoltseva. They were made of fleece of Tibetan goats and of saiga antelopes, executed in a complicated technique of double-faced weaving, in which the obverse and the reverse sides are indistinguishable. Unusually bright and colorful, they astounded contemporaries by the wealth of ornamental motifs and by the virtuosity of execution. Already at that time such shawls were valued very highly, and were sometimes priced at several thousand rubles. They became widely known and more than once were awarded medals in exhibitions.

A departure from the refined simplicity of the costumes of

the beginning of the century, already noticeable at the end of the first decade, became evident at the end of the 1810s through the 1820s. Dresses were shorter, losing their airiness; the silhouette became less severe and less plastic. The high waistline began to move lower, the corset reappeared, and both long sleeves with epaulets and short, lantern-shaped ones became fashionable. The skirt, cut on the bias at the sides and densely gathered at the back, acquired a bell silhouette, and was worn over a starched petticoat. The lightweight cottons were replaced by tightly woven silks, velvet, and wool. A more and more important role was played by the trimming of the dress: rolls, puffs, cordings, and flounces. Everyday dresses closely covered the body, while the ball gowns were often made of light muslin or tulle, and were generously decorated with garlands of large flowers, or with a rich bead, gold, or silver thread embroidery, or with polished steel plaquettes, for whose manufacture Tula's masters were famous in those years. Only the full-dress courtly gowns preserved the trains; they were made of tightly woven silk or velvet and decorated with embroidery in gilt thread, beaten gold lace, and spangles in a luxurious pattern made up of palmettes, meander, and other elements of the ornament of the Empire style.

During the end of the 18th and the first quarter of the 19th centuries an important place was occupied in the women's wardrobe by such kinds of outerwear as the spencer, a short jacket with long sleeves, usually lined for warmth with fur or cotton, and the redingote, which repeated the fashionable lines of the redingote dress.

In contrast to women's costume, that of men, beginning with the first decades of the 19th century, acquired a more severe, businesslike character and is of little interest from the artistic point of view.

Romanticism, so strikingly evident in Russian music, literature, and painting, did not bypass the fashion in dress. Women's dresses of the end of the 1820s and of the 1830s illustrate the newly formed "romantic" character of the costume. Its fanciful silhouette is defined by a skirt that became wider, a bodice with a "wasp" waistline, a low decolletage, and a sleeve densely gathered at the shoulder and tight at the wrist, that was named "gigot," or leg of mutton. Wide belts with large buckles became fashionable, often trimmed with faceted steel of Tula workmanship.

The new silhouette, new proportions, and new character of trimmings mark the woman's costume of the 1840s. Among the costumes of the period attention is attracted by the dress of pale, straw-colored faille, decorated with an original embroidery, the so-called "straw embroidery"—an example of the remarkable artistic achievement of anonymous women artisans.

During the 19th century the uniform coats of the Russian army and, most of all, those of the hussar regiments, were exceptionally colorful and decorative. Outstanding in their particular luxury were the gala gowns of the ladies at the court—"the ladies' dress uniforms," as A. S. Pushkin called them. The gowns shown in the exhibition belong to the second half of the 19th century, but they do repeat earlier examples created in accordance with a decree of 1834, which regulated strictly the cut, color, fabric, and character of the gold embroidery, depending on the wearer's rank at the court. These costumes preserve the cut of a dress with an opening in front, a skirt of white satin, a bodice with a deep decolletage, sleeves that can be folded back, and a very long train, whose length depended on the court rank of its owner. Dresses of green velvet with gold embroidery were worn by ladies in waiting and maids of honor, those of crimson velvet, by the maids of honor of the empress. These dresses are magnificent examples of Russian gold embroideries, which continued the traditions of the mastercraft of ancient Russia.

Ladies who were admitted to the court, but had no courtly rank, had to appear in dresses of the same style, but made of different fabric and with a different decoration. The gown was supplemented by a *kokoshnik* with a white veil. According to an apt remark of a contemporary, the costume reminded one of a "frenchified" sarafan.

Of special renown among the workshops that executed such gowns in the second half of the 19th century was the workshop in Saint Petersburg owned by O. N. Bulbenkova (Mme. Olga), which continued in operation through the beginning of the 20th century.

The mechanization of the textile industry in the second half of the 19th century made available to a wide circle of consumers dressy fabrics, machine-made laces, and embroideries. The appearance of the sewing machine reduced the cost of manufacture of clothing in Russia. The first shops of ready-made clothes were opened. A certain democratization of fashions began; nevertheless, the costumes of the wealthy remained as expensive as of old, and the trimming of fashionable women's dresses required painstaking handwork. The magnificent decoration of the morning dress made of white batiste embroidered overall in satin stitch is proof of the high quality of workmanship of the women embroiderers of the period.

As opposed to the 18th and the beginning of the 19th century, when the aristocracy was lawmaker of fashions in Russia, in the second half of the 19th century it was the rich bourgeoisie that claimed this role. Striving for a garish luxury led to an overloading of women's gowns with expensive fabrics, trimmings, and decorations. The fashion changed often, borrowing details from the costume of the years past, sometimes including them purely mechanically. In the 1850s and 60s, skirts were so wide that in order to preserve the fashionable silhouette a special construction of steel hoops fastened to each other by fabric tapes—the crinoline—was introduced. The choice of fabrics, the cut, and the decorations of the costume depended more and more on the purpose and the ownership of the costume. Very popular were all kinds of lace mantillas, mantlets, and shawls manufactured in workshops belonging to the landed gentry and located on their estates, as well as those embroidered in tambour stitch and with appliqués of batiste on tulle, for the execution of which the Russian women artisans were famous. The circular cape with a hood—the "burnoose"—a tribute to the enthusiasm for the Orient—became fashionable.

In the 1870s and 80s women's costume acquired more and more pretentious shapes, the crinoline was replaced by the "tournure" (bustle), over which the skirt was draped in the back, and in the 1880s the elongated bodice, very tightly laced at the waist and the enthusiam for assymetric draperies made their appearance. These costumes are distinguished by the use for one and the same dress of heavy fabrics of various textures, colors, and design: of plain and patterned satin, velvet, plush, as well as a wealth of drapings and the enthusiasm for lace trimmings, all kinds of fringes, and embroidery in glass beads and bugles. Such dresses fitted harmoniously into the interior decorations of the salons of those years, overloaded with furniture, upholstered in fabrics, with voluminous, massive folds in the draperies, and with a great number of fancifully molded frames.

The acknowledged lawmaker in the field of fashion at this period was the French dress designer F. Worth, who founded in 1857 in Paris the firm, which, up to the beginning of the 20th century, exerted an enormous influence on the development of the costume. He filled orders from Russian aristocracy as well. The dresses made by this firm shown in the exhibition are remarkable for their elegance and magnificent feeling for line and material.

At the end of the 19th century and the beginning of the 20th century Russian designers in Petersburg—Brisac, A. T. Ivanova, and A. G. Gindus—gained recognition. In particular one must note the work done by N. Lamanova, who opened a workshop in 1885 in Moscow. A unique collection in the Hermitage of costumes made by this remarkable dressmaker makes it possible to show the work of various periods of her activity.

A great influence began to be exerted on the fashion of the end of the 19th and the beginning of the 20th century by the emancipation of women, their participation in public and work life, and the enthusiasm for sport. It became necessary to create a comfortable costume. In the following years a further simplification of clothing took place, the difference between the modest day dress and the dressy evening gown becoming still more pronounced. One of the characteristics of the evening gowns of this period was the combination of heavy fabrics—velvet, satin, brocade—with the semitransparent ones —gauze, chiffon, and lace—and the abundance of embroideries in glass beads, bugles, strass, spangles, and gilt thread.

Among the fashion designers of that period, Paul Poiret in Paris, a courageous innovator in the field of fashion, was greatly influenced by the performances in Paris of the Russian ballet, with settings and costumes designed by L. Bakst and A. Benoit.

Samples of clothing worn in Russia before the first World War complete the exhibition of Russian urban costume. In the post-war years was formed the new contemporary character of clothing. This new character was closer to our present-day shapes than to the costume of the beginning of the century, but this is already a new epoch in the development of this branch of art.

The organizers of the exhibition hope that it will arouse interest in a wide circle of visitors, will be useful and interesting for the specialists, will permit the public to become better acquainted with the history of our people, and, as a final result, will contribute to the further rapprochement between the people of U.S.S.R. and the U.S.A.

L. EFIMOVA, Historical Museum
T. KORSHUNOVA, The Hermitage
L. EFREMOVA

CATALOGUE

Russian Costume from the 11th to the 17th Century

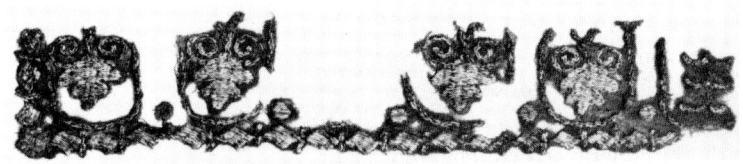

1

1. Fragment of Collar
   Silk embroidered with gold thread. From an 11th-century burial mound. Vladimir region, village of Davydkovo.
   Inv. No. 55421 op. 1068-351. Acquired in 1924.
   Historical Museum, Moscow

2. Fragment of Collar
   Silk embroidered with gold thread. From a 12th-century woman's burial mound near St. John's Church, Smolensk.
   Inv. No. 102293 op. 2101-1. Acquired in 1972.
   Historical Museum

3-4. Fragments of a Woven Gold Band
   From a 12th-century burial mound. Vladimir region, village of Shushpanovo.
   Inv. No. 78605 ot. 999-1,2. Acquired in 1937.
   Historical Museum

5-9. Three Fragments of Silk Fabrics
   Woven and embroidered with gold threads and silk. From a mid-12th-century burial mound. The Assumption Cathedral of the Moscow Kremlin.
   Excavations of 1967, burial 28, Nos. 31,32,45.
   Kremlin Museums, Moscow

10. **Fragment of Wool Cloth**
    From an 11th-century burial mound. Kaluga region, village of Dobroselye.
    Inv. No. 25778 op. 234-75. Acquired in 1892.
    Historical Museum

11- **Fragments of Wool Cloth with Printed Design**
12. From an 11th-century burial mound. Chernigov region, village of Levinki.
    Inv. No. 76990 op. 793-32,33. Acquired in 1934.
    Historical Museum

13. **Fragment of Printed Wool Cloth**
    With ornament designs worked in colored threads. From a 12th-century burial mound. Moscow region, village of Bolshevo.
    Inv. No. 42044 op. 446-16. Acquired in 1904.
    Historical Museum

14. **Fragment of Wool Cloth**
    From a 12th-century burial mound. Smolensk region, village of Kokhany.
    Inv. No. 25778 op. 219-458. Acquired in 1892.
    Historical Museum

15. **Fragment of Wool Cloth**
    With a woven design. From a 12th-century burial mound. Smolensk region.
    Inv. No. 42796 op. 202-540. Acquired in 1894.
    Historical Museum

16. **Kolt** (woman's ornament worn on the temple)
    Granulated silver. Place of the find unknown. 12th-early 13th century.
    Inv. No. 41425 op. 1952/2. Acquired in 1894.
    Historical Museum

17. **Ring Worn on the Temple**
    Gold. Three beads. From the treasure trove found near Kiev. 12th-early 13th century.

Inv. No. 76990 op. $\frac{2111}{6}$. Acquired in 1934.
Historical Museum

18. **Ring Worn on the Temple**
Gold. Three beads. From the treasure trove found on the territory of the Tithe Church in Kiev. 12th-13th century.
Inv. No. 54746 op. $\frac{2214}{4}$. Acquired in 1924.
Historical Museum

19. **Ring Worn on the Temple**
Gold. Three beads. From the treasure trove found near Kiev. 12th-early 13th century.
Inv. No. 76990 op. $\frac{2111}{8}$. Acquired in 1934.
Historical Museum

20- **Rings Worn on the Temple**
21. Silver. Openwork. From the treasure trove found near Kiev. 12th-early 13th century.
Inv. No. 76990 op. $\frac{1673}{88,90}$. Acquired in 1934.
Historical Museum

22. **Ring Worn on the Temple**
Silver gilt. Three beads. From the treasure trove found near Kiev.
Inv. No. 43078 op. $\frac{1734}{4}$. Acquired in 1905.
Historical Museum

23. **Ring Worn on the Temple**
Silver gilt. Three beads. From the treasure trove found near Kiev. 12th-early 13th century.
Inv. No. 43080 op. $\frac{1734}{6}$. Acquired in 1905.
Historical Museum

24. **Ring Worn on the Temple**
Silver. Diamond-shaped. From a 12th-century burial mound. Moscow region, village of Aseyevo.
Inv. No. 69665 op. $\frac{442}{1}$. Acquired in 1924.
Historical Museum

25- **Rings Worn on the Temple**
28. Low-standard silver. Seven-flanged blade. From a 12th-century burial mound. Moscow region, village of Puzikovo.
    Inv. No. 56112 op. 409/46-47-48-49. Acquired in 1934.
    Historical Museum

29- **Rings Worn on the Temple**
30. Low-standard silver. Spiral-shaped. From an 11th-century burial mound. Kursk region, Belogorsko-Nikolayevsky Monastery.
    Inv. No. 76990 op. $\frac{773}{97-98}$. Acquired in 1934.
    Historical Museum

31- **Rings Worn on the Temple**
37. Low-standard silver. Bracelet form. From an 11th-12th-century burial mound. Kaluga region, village of Kurganye.
    Inv. No. 42215 op. $\frac{259}{31-37}$. Acquired in 1904.
    Historical Museum

38- **Rings Worn on the Temple**
44. Silver. Early 13th century. From the Belevsky treasure trove. Tula region.
    Inv. No. 26631-37 op. $\frac{226}{4-10}$. Acquired in 1891.
    Historical Museum

45. **Neck Ornament**
    Silver. From a 12th-century burial mound. Moscow region, village of Aniskino.
    Inv. No. 78607 op. $\frac{435}{4}$. Acquired in 1937.
    Historical Museum

46. **Neck Ornament**
    Bronze. From an 11th-century burial mound. Chernigov region, village of Vlazovichi.
    Inv. No. N32884 688/9.
    Historical Museum

47. **Neck Ornament**
    Bronze. From an 11th-century burial mound. Chernigov region.

Inv. No. 32884 op. 718/12. Acquired in 1895.
Historical Museum

48. **Neck Ornament**
 11th century. Chernigov region, village of Mamekovo.
 Inv. No. 46042 op. 2192/1. Acquired in 1910.
 Historical Museum

49. **Beads**
 Carnelian and cut glass. From a 12th-century burial mound. Kaluga region, village of Dobroselye.
 Inv. No. 25778 op. 234/68-70. Acquired in 1892.
 Historical Museum

50. **Beads**
 Glass with gold spacers. From an 11th-century burial mound. Kaluga region, village of Kolchino.
 Inv. No. 22215 220-3. Acquired in 1904.
 Historical Museum

51. **Beads**
 Blue glass. Variously shaped. From an 11th-century burial mound. Vladimir region.
 Inv. No. 54746 op. 2194/1324. Acquired in 1924.
 Historical Museum

52. **Beads**
 Gold and glass. From an 11th-century burial mound. Vladimir region.
 Inv. No. 54746 2194/1267.
 Historical Museum

53. **Beads**
 Colored glass and stones. From a 12th-century burial mound. Vladimir region.
 Inv. No. 54746 2194/1327.
 Historical Museum

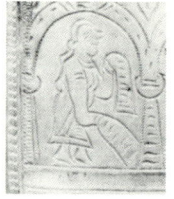

54

54. Bracelet
Silver and silver gilt with engraved ornamentation. Two-hinged. 12th-early 13th century.
Inv. No. 54746 2103-1 SB-1360.
Historical Museum

55. Bracelet
Silver. Woven from six wires. 12th-early 13th century. Kiev region.
Inv. No. 25517 1916-1 SB-17120.
Historical Museum

56. Bracelet
Silver. Woven and twisted with flattened ends. 12th century. Kiev region.
Inv. No. 43629 1917-1.
Historical Museum

57- Two Bracelets
58. Twisted silver. From the treasure trove found on the territory of the Tithe Church in Kiev. 12th-13th century.
Inv. No. 54746 op. 2214/5-6. Acquired in 1924.
Historical Museum

59- Two Rings
60. Silver decorated with niello. From the treasure trove found near the village of Shmarovo, Kaluga region.
Inv. No. 78605 op. 1063/2,4. Acquired in 1937.
Historical Museum

Dress with straw embroidery (347)

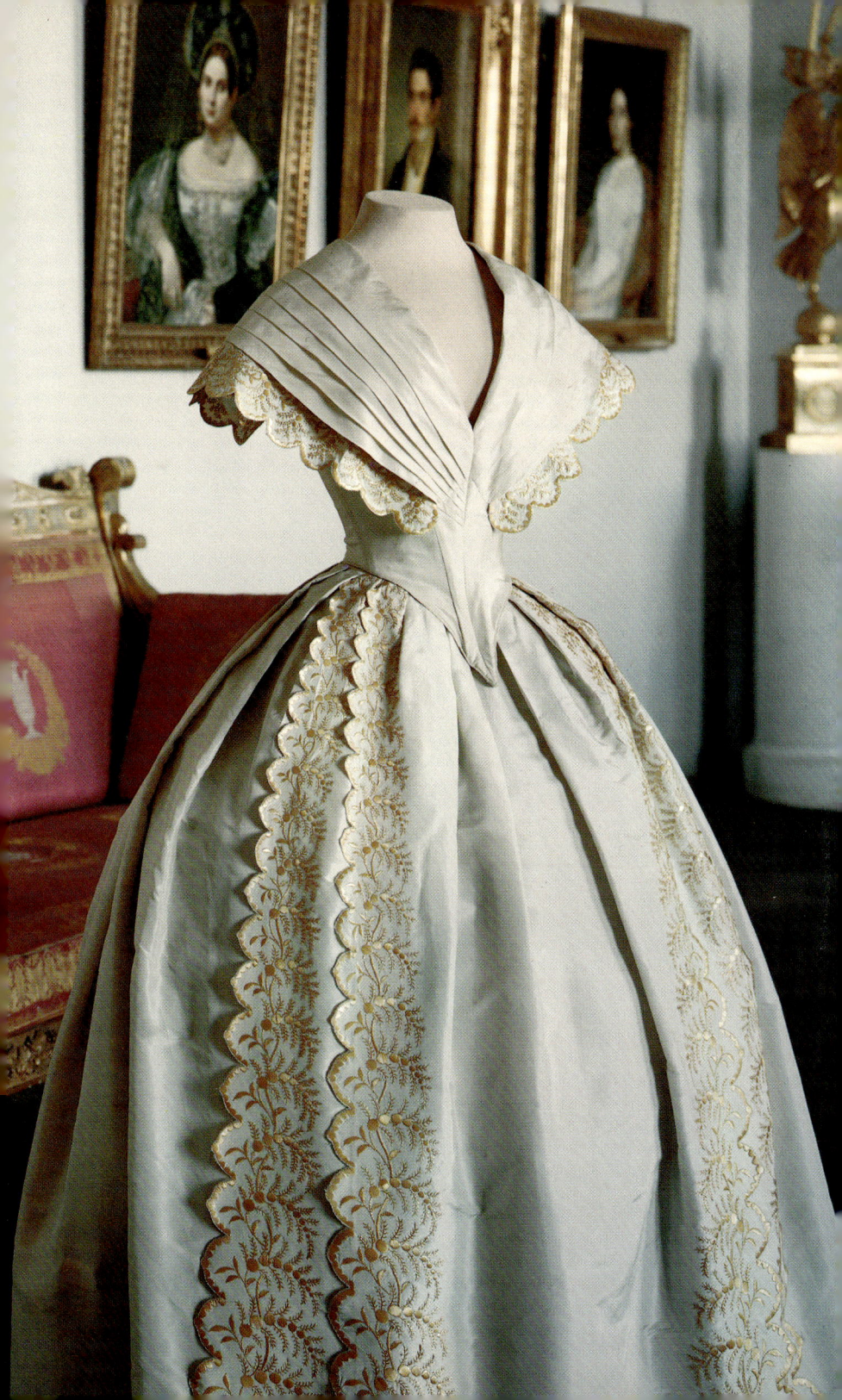

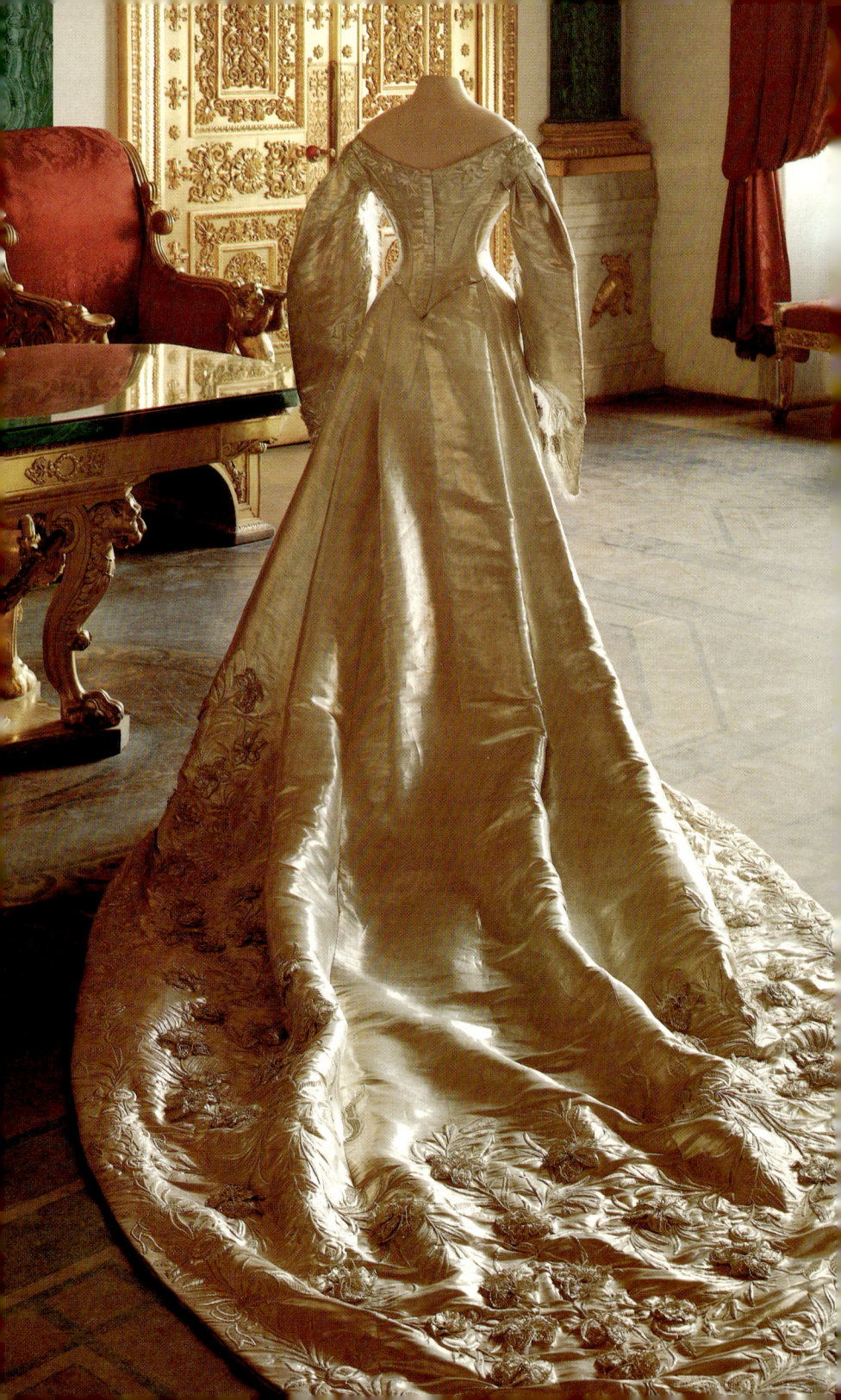

61. **Woman's Headdress**
 Crown of braided gold threads, the hard front of silk satin decorated with embroidery. The design in the form of diamonds and crosses is worked in gold thread. Belonged to Tsarina Anastasiya Romanovna. 1560 (?). Moscow.
 Inv. No. 36656. Found during the restoration work of the Ascension Cathedral of the Moscow Kremlin in 1929.
 Kremlin Museums

62. **Okhaben** (woman's outer garment)
 Golden silk corded material. Open, with side panels cut on the bias with slits up the sides. Long-sleeved, decorated with gold galloon. The fabric was manufactured in western Europe, 17th century. First half of the 17th century. Russian work.
 Inv. No. 98674 B-2617. Acquired in 1964.
 Historical Museum

63. **Woman's High Boot**
 Red velvet. High-heeled, with wide calf. Leather sole. Decorated with embroidery worked in pearls. Second half of the 17th century. Moscow.
 Inv. okhr. No. 4031. The main collection of the Armory.
 Kremlin Museums

64. **Shirinka** (handkerchief)
 White taffeta with white openwork worked in gold threads and pearls. Russian work.
 Inv. okhr. No. 13242. Patriarch's Sacristy.
 Kremlin Museums

65. **Gloves** (pair)
 Knitted dark purple silk. Bell-shaped at the wrist. Decorated with gold embroidery, silver bone lace, and pearls. 17th century. England (?).
 Inv. okhr. No. 4035. The main collection of the Armory.
 Kremlin Museums

Court dress (402)

66. **Caftan** (long field tunic)
Russian *bois de rose* silk "baiberek" manufactured at the factory of Zakhary Pavlov. Full-length, open, with side panels cut on the bias with slits up the sides, and wide sleeves. Decorated with 17th-century western European gold lace. Worn by Peter I.
Inv. okhr. No. 144. The main collection of the Armory.
Kremlin Museums

67. **Staff**
Silver gilt. In the form of a walking stick, decorated with eagles' heads, with a figured staff head. Ornamented with chased designs and precious stones. 17th century. Moscow.
Inv. okhr. No. 104. The main collection of the Armory.
Kremlin Museums

68. **Rubakha** (boy's shirt)
White cotton. Tuniclike, with straight short sleeves, and an inset of red taffeta in the underpart of the sleeve. Opens at the neck, with a slit to the left of center. Decorated with embroidery worked with couched gold thread. Geometric design. 17th century. Russian work.
Inv. No. 56746 B-144. Acquired in 1925.
Historical Museum

69. **Fragment of the Rubakha Worn by Dmitry Pozharsky**
Decorated on the shoulders. Gold thread is laid in rows and couched down with the same thread on the silk background.
Inv. No. 53594, V-296. Acquired in 1922.
Historical Museum

70. **Seafarer's Caftan**
Homespun broadcloth. Open, with side panels cut on the bias and slits up the sides. The chest is decorated with six rows of strips on each panel. From the excavations of an archaeological expedition on the Taimyr Peninsula. Reconstruction. First quarter of the 17th century. Russian work.
Inv. No. NV-5123. Acquired in 1946.
Historical Museum

71. **Ryasa** (housecoat)
    Dark blue velvet with a vegetative design. Open, with a row of buttons down the front, wide sleeves, and a little standing collar. 1650s. Russian work. The fabric was manufactured in Italy, mid-17th century. Worn by Patriarch Nikon (1652–1658).
    Inv. okhr. No. 13181 op. 12132. Patriarch's Sacristy.
    Kremlin Museums

72. **Stikhar** (robe worn in religious ceremonies)
    Brocade with a large vegetative ornament. The shoulder is of purple velvet and decorated with embroidery worked in pearls, gold thread, and sequins. Back of sleeves and skirt are trimmed with gold bone lace. The cross is decorated with pearls and emeralds set in gold. 17th century. Russian work. The fabric was manufactured in Italy, 17th century.
    Inv. okhr. No. 13109 op. 12059.
    Kremlin Museums

73. **Felon** (robe worn in religious ceremonies)
    Pink brocade with a large vegetative ornament. The shoulders are of black velvet decorated with a vegetative design worked in pearls, with gold discs, rubies, emeralds, and sapphires. The tunic is of blue silk decorated with gold bone lace. Late 17th century. Russian work. The brocade was imported from France.
    Inv. okhr. No. 16154 op. 16234.
    Kremlin Museums

74- **Strips with a Button** (two pairs)
75. Braided gold and silver threads. Tassels at the ends. Buttons are round and covered with cloth. 17th century. Moscow.
    Inv. okhr. No. 4019, okhr. No. 4020. The main collection of the Armory.
    Kremlin Museums

76. **Button**
    Silver. Composed of two hemispheres, decorated with a chased design representing circles and petals. The technique employs granulation and little round cuts. Crowned with a pyramidlike

granulation. 17th century. Russian work. Size: 4.3 x 8.2 cm.
Inv. No. 11537 shch/ok 21621 SB-9493. Acquired in 1905.
Historical Museum

77. **Button**
Silver gilt. Large, almond-shaped, and composed of two spheres with a chased scale design. The loop is surrounded by a chased design in the form of a twelve-petal rosette. 17th century. Russian work. Size: 5.5 x 3.3 x 2.7 cm.
Inv. No. 11290 shch/ok 7509 SB-7190. Acquired in 1905.
Historical Museum

78. **Button**
Silver gilt. Egg-shaped. Solidly covered with etched design. First half of the 17th century. Moscow. Size: 7.3 x 5.5 cm.
Inv. No. 75701/ok 8479 SB-2954. Acquired in 1933.
Historical Museum

79. **Button**
Silver gilt. Spherical. Completely decorated with granulation set with rings. 17th century. Russian work. Length: 4.7 cm.
Inv. No. 86913/ok 7424 SB-2923.
Historical Museum

80. **Button**
Solid silver, with multicolored enamel and plated silver stars. 17th century. Russia. Size: 3.5 x 2.4 x 2.4 cm.
Inv. No. 75701/ok 8322 SV-4066. Acquired in 1953.
Historical Museum

81. **Button**
Solid silver. Openwork, decorated with an intricate design of filigree and granulation. 17th century. Russia. Size: 4.9 x 3.3 x 3.3 cm.
Inv. No. 50489/ok 21622 SB-9495. Acquired in 1917.
Historical Museum

82. **Button**
Silver gilt. Spherical. Openwork, filigree ornament solidly cov-

ered with granulation. Granulated silver beads form a pyramid. 17th century. Russia. Size: 3.1 x 1.9 x 1.8 cm.
Inv. No. 35503/ok 21635 SB-10026. Acquired in 1898.
Historical Museum

83. **Button**
Silver gilt. Pear-shaped. Solidly covered with filigree ornament and painted enamel with plated silver stars and beads. A crowned red stone at the end. Mid-17th century. Moscow. Size: 3 x 2.2 cm.
Inv. No. 75701/47 ok 8367 SB-4067. Acquired in 1933.
Historical Museum

84. **Button**
Silver with traces of gilt. Spherical. With an ornament of embossed circles in a leafy setting. 17th-18th century. Russia. Size: 5 x 3.3 x 3.1 cm.
Inv. No. 39135/ok 21623 SB-10005. Acquired in 1901.
Historical Museum

85. **Button**
Silver gilt. Pear-shaped. Openwork, ornamented with five filigree rose petals covered with granulation. At the end is a rosette with five petals and granulation soldered to the silverwork. Late 17th-early 18th century. Russia. From the P.I. Shchukin collection of 1905.
Inv. No. 19129 shch/ok 21823 SB-9406.
Historical Museum

86. **Button**
Silver gilt. Pear-shaped. Openwork. Back is ornamented with six round petals of filigree with plated silver flowers and a silver bead at the center. Late 17th-early 18th century. Russia. Length: 3.3 cm.
Inv. No. 53492/ok 21825 SB 9407.
Historical Museum

41

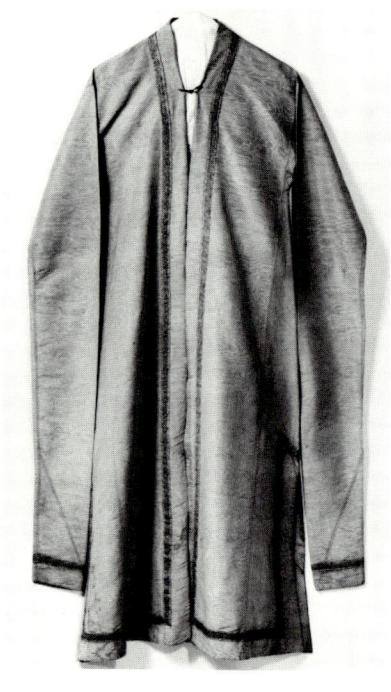

62

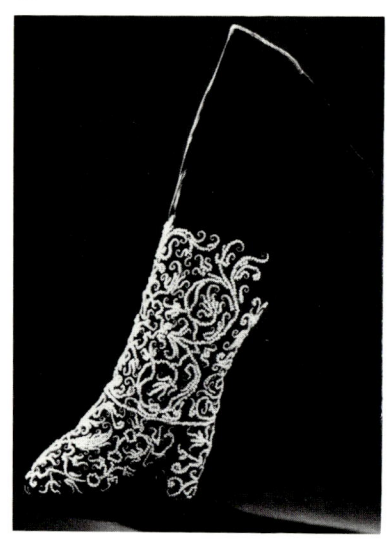

63

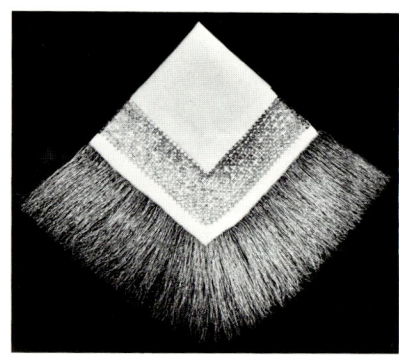

64

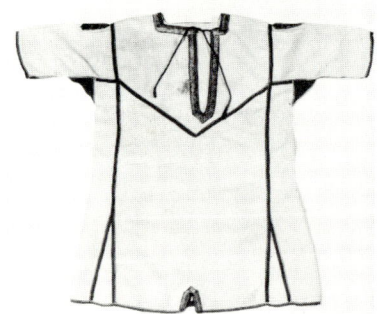

68

66

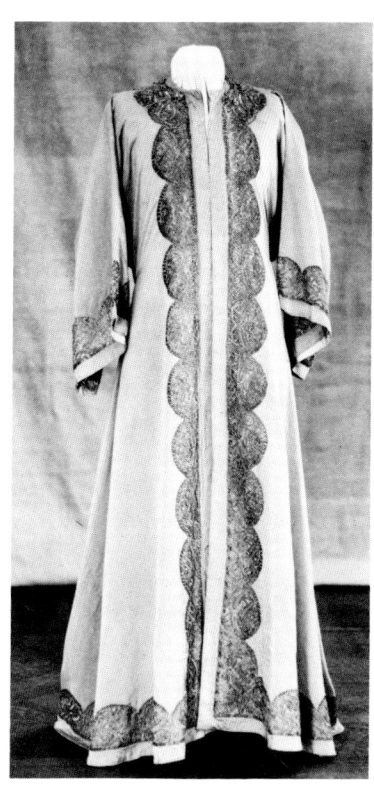

77, 78, 80, 83, 84

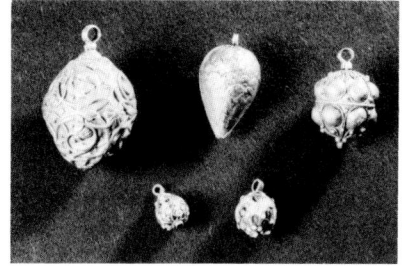

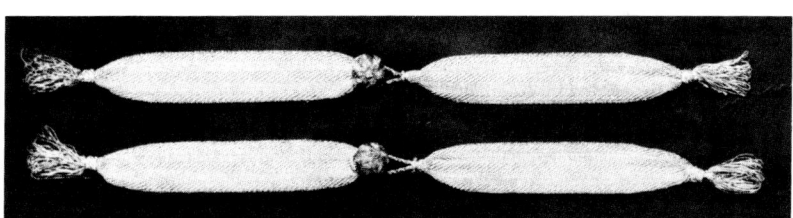

74, 75

87. **Button**
Silver. Spherical, composed of two hemispheres. Openwork, decorated with granulation. Five large silver beads form a pyramid. 17th-18th century. Russia. Size: 3.7 x 2.5 x 2.5 cm.
Inv. No. 50489/ok 21630 SB-9486. Acquired in 1917.
Historical Museum

88. **Earrings** (pair)
Silver with carnelian pendants. 16th century. Russia. Length: 7.8 cm.
Inv. No. 12962 shch/ok 21239 SB-7312. Acquired in 1905.
Historical Museum

89. **Earrings** (pair)
Silver. The pendants are decorated with beads and flat, stylized figures of birds. 16th-17th century. Russia. Length: 7.3 cm.
Inv. No. 12713 shch/ok 21335 SV-7475. Acquired in 1905.
Historical Museum

90. **Earrings** (pair)
Two silver rods with rosettes and glass beads. 16th-17th century. Russia. Length: 8 cm.
Inv. No. 12730 shch/ok 21337 SV-8817. Acquired in 1905.
Historical Museum

91. **Earrings** (pair)
Silver gilt. Two openwork silver beads in each earring. 16th-17th century. Russia. Size: 3.8 x 2 cm.
Inv. No. 17996/ok 21339 SB-11544. Acquired in 1891.
Historical Museum

92. **Earrings** (pair)
Silver gilt. Floral motif with an ornament in the form of two birds. Executed in the old Russian tradition. 18th century. Russia. Size: 4.6 x 2.6 cm.
Inv. No. 54679/ok 21352 SB-12026.
Historical Museum

93. **Earrings** (pair)
Silver gilt. Three silver gilt rods decorated with mother-of-pearl beads and glass attached to a loop of thick wire. Executed in the old tradition. 18th century. Russia. Size: 4.3 cm.
  Inv. No. 16151/ok 21383 SV-7264.
  Historical Museum

94. **Cross on a Chain**
Solid silver. Links shaped like two figure eights are joined by spacer rings. 17th century. Russia. Size of the cross: 7.6 x 6.8 cm. Length of chain: 100 cm.
  Inv. No. 67591/8 ok 15769 SB-1817. Acquired in 1829.
  Historical Museum

95. **Cross on a Chain**
Solid silver. 17th-18th century. Novgorod. Size of the cross: 8.2 x 7 cm. Length of chain: 99 cm.
  Inv. No. 35302/ok 7761 SB-2862. Acquired in 1898.
  Historical Museum

96. **Sample of Gold Embroidery**
Vegetative design on black velvet background.
  Inv. No. 20305 shch RB-241. Acquired in 1905.
  Historical Museum

97. **Sample of Gold Embroidery**
Vegetative motif and birds on red velvet background.
  Inv. No. 19830 shch RB-209. Acquired in 1905.
  Historical Museum

98. **Oplechye** (robe worn during religious ceremonies)
Gold embroidery on red velvet background. Vegetative design. Late 17th-early 18th century. Russia.
  Inv. No. 55753 V-4. Acquired in 1924.
  Historical Museum

99. **Sample of Gold Embroidery**
Red velvet. Design represents trees, griffins, and birds. Late 17th-early 18th century. Russia.
  Inv. No. 19764 shch RB-339. Acquired in 1905.
  Historical Museum

100. Printed Cloth
    Homespun linen canvas. Printed with vegetative design. 17th century. Russia.
    Inv. No. 67012 A-4144. Acquired in 1928.
    Historical Museum

101. Printed Cloth
    Homespun linen canvas. Printed with vegetative design and ornamental motifs. 17th century. Russia.
    Inv. No. 38510 Kr. B-73. Acquired in 1900.
    Historical Museum

102. Printed Cloth
    Homespun linen canvas. Oriental print. 17th century. Russia.
    Inv. No. 37125 Kr. B-21. Acquired in 1899.
    Historical Museum

Folk Costume from the 18th to the Early 20th Century

Woman's Holiday Dress
Second half of the 18th century. Central Russia.

103. SARAFAN Pink silk with a woven multicolored floral pattern. Panels cut on the bias, opening with a row of buttons down the front. Decorated with strips of gold galloon.
    Inv. No. 57991 B-426 SV-1413. Acquired in 1926.

104. RUBAKHA White cambric. Long, with straight panels and long wide sleeves gathered at the wrist. Embroidered floral sprays are worked with white thread in chain stitch.
    Inv. No. 82898 B-1217. Acquired in 1949.

105. BELT Gold galloon decorated with tassels at the ends.
    Inv. No. 87833 I-578. Acquired in 1953.
    Historical Museum

Woman's Holiday Dress
Late 18th century. Central Russia.
106. SARAFAN Blue ribbed silk brocaded in multicolored floral design. Panels cut on the bias, opening with a row of buttons down the front. Trimmed with gold galloon.
Inv. No. 50455 B-51 SV-1417. Acquired in 1917.
107. DUSHEGREYA (lined jacket) Red brocade. Short, with closefitting waist, low set-in sleeves, and turndown collar. Decorated with gold galloon and embroidered in gold thread.
Inv. No. 36753 B-523. Acquired in 1895.
Historical Museum

Woman's Holiday Dress
Late 18th century. Northern Russia.
108. SARAFAN Purple silk with sprays and borders brocaded in multicolored thread. Panels cut on the bias, opening with a row of buttons down the front. Trimmed with gold bone lace and colored tinsel.
Inv. No. 78014 B-651 SV1419. Acquired in 1936.
109. RUBAKHA (shirt) Blue silk with a woven vegetative design; incorporates pieces of printed cotton fabric. Short with straight panels and long sleeves tightening at the wrist.
Inv. No. 55753 B-1002. Acquired in 1924.
110. CHEST ORNAMENT Mother-of-pearl and glass in metal.
Inv. No. 37212 Ch-225. Acquired in 1899.
Historical Museum

Woman's Holiday Dress
18th century. Central Russia.
111. SARAFAN Pink silk with floral pattern worked in multicolored threads. Panels cut on the bias, opening with a row of buttons down the front.
Inv. No. 54768 B-422 SV-1416. Acquired in 1924.
112. DUSHEGREYA (lined jacket) White silk patterned with gold thread. Short, long-sleeved, collarless. Tight-fitting, with a short skirtlike box-and-inverted pleat continuation of the bodice at the back. Decorated with silver fringe.
Inv. No. 102108 B-3297. Acquired in 1971.
Historical Museum

Woman's Holiday Dress
Late 18th-early 19th century. Nizhny Novgorod.
113. SARAFAN Purple red brocade. Panels cut on the bias, opening with a row of buttons down the front. Decorated with gold galloon.
Inv. No. 95085 B-1929. Acquired in 1957.
114. RUBAKHA (shirt) White cambric with sprays and leaves embroidered in white thread. The design is worked in chain-stitch. Long, with tight, long, low, set-in sleeves slashed at the wrist.
Inv. No. 89401 b 2145b.
115. EPANECHKA (short mantle) Red velvet. Padded with flax tow. Short with shoulder straps, pleated. The background is solidly embroidered with couched gold and silver thread.
Inv. No. 75303 69632 b-347. Acquired in 1933.
116. PLATOK (kerchief) Purple taffeta, solidly embroidered with gold. Size: 91 x 89 cm.
Inv. No. 42567 D-626. Acquired in 1905.
Historical Museum

Woman's Holiday Dress
Late 18th-early 19th century. Vladimir region.
117. SARAFAN Purple damask with floral pattern worked in gold and silver thread. Trimmed with metallic bone lace.
Inv. No. ERT-7208. Acquired in 1941.
118. DUSHEGREYA (lined jacket) Brocade. Gold embroidery on silver background.
Inv. No. ERT-7287. Acquired in 1941.
The Hermitage, Leningrad

Maiden's Holiday Dress
First half of the 19th century. Northern Russia, Kargopol.
119. RUBAKHA (shirt) Homespun linen canvas. Long, with straight wide sleeves gathered at the wrist. Decorated with a woven pattern and embroidery worked with multicolored silk and sequins in various stitches.
Inv. No. 42343 B-974. Acquired in 1904.
120. BELT Homespun wool.
Inv. No. 101275/79 I-735. Acquired in 1969.
Historical Museum

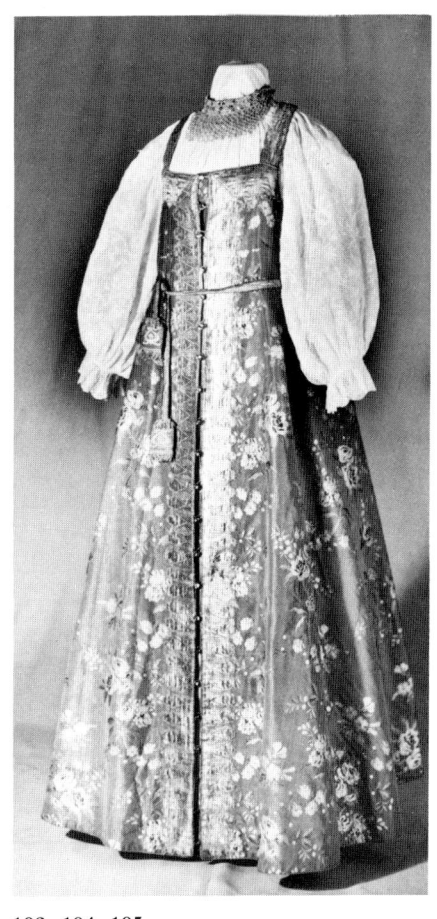 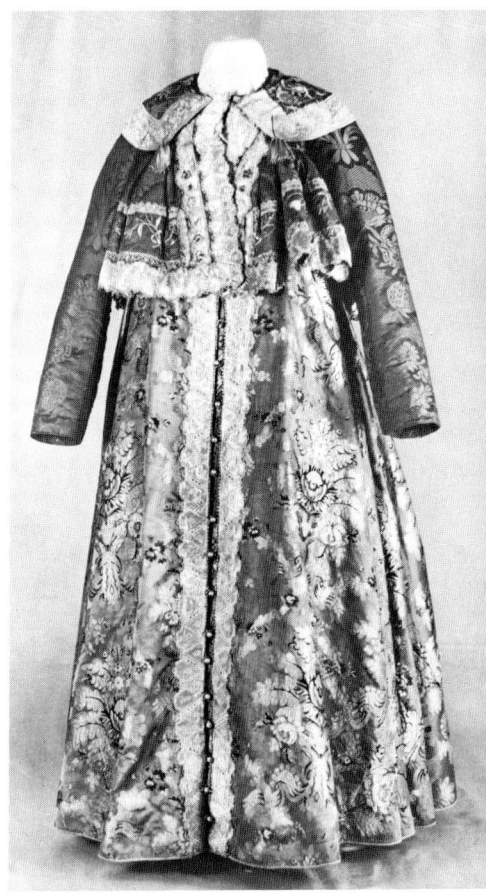

103, 104, 105   106, 107

Female Peasant's Holiday Dress
19th century. Vologda region.

121. SARAFAN Homespun printed linen. White-outlined vegetative design worked with orange polka dots on a blue ground. Cut straight and held up by narrow straps. Decorated with pieces of calico and colored wool thread.
Inv. No. 57987 B-460. Acquired in 1926.

122. RUBAKHA Homespun linen canvas. Short. Embroidered in multicolored silk and flax worked in stem and darning stitches.
Inv. No. 54019 B-973. Acquired in 1922.

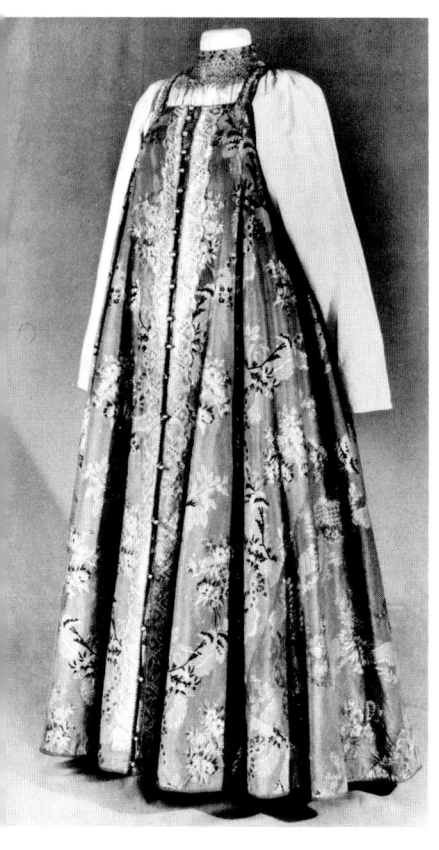 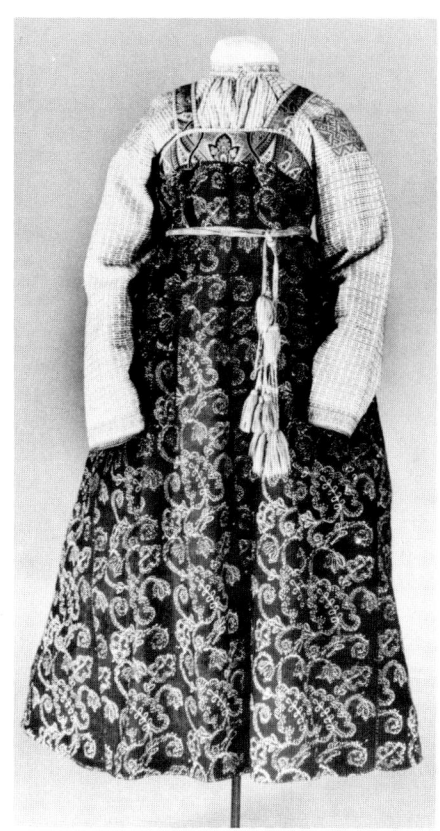

111 125, 126, 127

123. PEREDNIK (apron) Homespun linen canvas. Long, with a little flap in front above the waistline to cover the chest. Embroidered with red linen thread worked in cross stitch and decorated with knitted lace.
Inv. No. 53142 B-1017. Acquired in 1922.

124. OZHERELOK (necklace) Narrow strips of linen canvas decorated with mother-of-pearl and colored glass.
Inv. No. 77649 Ch-112. Acquired in 1935.
Historical Museum

Female Peasant's Dress
Late 19th-early 20th century. Vologda region, Solvychegodsk.
125. SARAFAN Homespun printed linen. White-outlined pattern on a blue background. Panels cut on the bias, with a vertical seam down the front. Decorated with pieces of calico and braided bands.
Inv. No. 101275 B-2966. Acquired in 1969.
126. RUBAKHA Homespun linen with red pattern. Short.
Inv. No. 101275 B-2971. Acquired in 1969.
127. BELT Braided wool, with fringes at the ends.
Inv. No. 101275 I-736. Acquired in 1969.
128. SAMSHURA (headdress) Red calico. The front is decorated with gold embroidery.
Inv. No. 101275 Ye-1002. Acquired in 1969.
Historical Museum

Female Peasant's Dress
Early 20th century. Arkhangelsk region.
129. SARAFAN Multicolored homespun cloth. Cut straight, held up by straps.
130. RUBAKHA Multicolored homespun cloth. Short, with straight panels and wide long sleeves gathered at the wrist. Decorated with red calico and braided band.
131. POYAS (belt) Homespun wool.
Inv. No. 101275 B-2995 a, b, v. Acquired in 1969.
Historical Museum

Young Peasant Girl's Dress
Early 20th century. Northern Russia.
132. RUBAKHA Made of two panels of cloth. The upper is red calico, the lower is homespun linen. The hem is bordered by a strip of red embroidery.
Inv. No. 83206 B-1361. Acquired in 1950.
133. BELT Braided wool.
Inv. No. 54752 I-488. Acquired in 1950.
134. FILLET Red silk. Embroidered with gold threads couched down in rows. Decorated with tinsel.
Inv. No. 48070 Kr. B-613. Acquired in 1912.
Historical Museum

Female Peasant's Two-Piece Holiday Dress
Late 19th-early 20th century. Arkhangelsk region.
135. SKIRT Golden silk patterned fabric. Cut straight, gathered at the waist. The hem is bordered by a strip of red cashmere.
136. KAZACHOK (topshirt) Golden silk patterned fabric, the same as the skirt No. 135. High collar with wide sleeves gathered on the shoulders and tight at the wrist, with a row of buttons in front. Tight-fitting, with a skirtlike pleated continuation of the bodice at the back.
   Inv. No. 83206 a,b 1368 a,b.
137. SCARF Tan lace. Handwork. Vologda.
   Inv. No. 85657 Z-1096/235.
   Historical Museum

138. **Maiden's Rubakha**
   Two panels of different material. The upper part is of red patterned silk damask manufactured in Russia in the 18th century; the lower part is of white homespun linen. Embroidered in dark red with geometric pattern. First half of the 19th century. Northern Russia.
   Inv. No. 96430 173 B-2285. Acquired in 1959.
   Historical Museum

Holiday Dress of a Urals Cossack Woman
Second half of the 19th century. Russia.
139. SARAFAN Blue patterned silk. Panels cut on the bias, opening in front. Decorated with gold galloon and rock crystal buttons.
   Inv. No. E/rt-10239, a.
140. RUBAKHA White patterned fabric, blue satin, and calico. Embroidered in gold thread worked in chain and satin stitches and decorated with gold galloon.
   Inv. No. E/rt-10239 b.
141. BELT Gold galloon.
   Inv. No. E/rt-15146. Acquired in 1941.
   The Hermitage

Holiday Dress of a Urals Cossack Woman
Late 19th century.
142. RUBAKHA White silk satin, embroidered in metal threads.
   Inv. No. 79846B 686/3. Acquired in 1938.

143. SARAFAN Lavender gray silk. Panels cut on the bias, open, with a row of buttons down the front. Gold galloon.
Inv. No. 79846B 686/4. Acquired in 1938.
144. BELT Gold galloon. Tassels at the ends.
Inv. No. 79846B 686/2. Acquired in 1938.
Historical Museum

Female Peasant's Dress
Mid-19th century. Kalinin region.
145. SARAFAN Red cotton. Panels cut on the bias. Opening with buttons down the front. Trimmed with patterned bands.
Inv. No. 102785/1 B-3351
146. RUBAKHA Bleached linen canvas with insets of red calico. Short, with straight panels.
Inv. No. 102785/2 B-3352. Acquired in 1968.
147. BELT Gold galloon.
Inv. No. GIM 83206 i 547. Acquired in 1968.
Historical Museum

Female Peasant's Holiday Dress
Mid-19th century. Moscow region.
148. SARAFAN Dark blue cotton. Panels cut on the bias, opening with a row of buttons down the front.
Inv. No. 58451 B-474a.
149. RUBAKHA Calico. Sleeves are solidly worked in strips of red embroidery and braided gold.
Inv. Nos. 58451 B-474 b. Acquired in 1926.
150. PEREDNIK (apron) Cashmere decorated with strips of woven pattern and bands.
Inv. No. 98598 B-2664. Acquired in 1964.
Historical Museum

Female Peasant's Holiday Dress
Late 19th-early 20th century. Smolensk region.
151. RUBAKHA Homespun linen canvas. Long, one-piece cut, with straight panels. Sleeves are made of red woven panels and embroidery worked in multicolored thread.
Inv. No. 96331 B-2331 a.

152. SARAFAN Blue cotton. Panels cut on the bias, false buttons down the front. Decorated with silk patterned ribbon, a strip of red calico, tinsel, and a white band.
Inv. No. 96331 B-2331 v.
153. BELT Multicolored wool with fringes at the ends.
Inv. No. 54752 KrB-10. Acquired in 1959.
Historical Museum

Female Peasant's Holiday Dress
Early 20th century. Smolensk region.
154. PONEVA (skirt) Checkered homespun wool with an inset of blue cotton fabric and red calico.
Inv. No. 95947/66 b-2141.
155. RUBAKHA Homespun linen canvas. Short, with straight panels and frilled collar.
Inv. No. 83920 B1576.
156. APRON Homespun linen canvas. Sleeveless. Shaped bodice. Trimmed with red calico, patterned cotton, and stitching in a geometric pattern.
Inv. No. 83925 B 1581. Acquired in 1950.
Historical Museum

Female Peasant's Dress
Last quarter of the 19th century. Ryazan region.
157. RUBAKHA Homespun linen canvas. Short. Decorated with strips of red calico, blue and yellow cotton, and embroidery worked in cross-stitch. Sleeves are gathered at the wrist forming a frill.
Inv. No. 55856 B-976. Acquired in 1924.
158. PONEVA (skirt) Blue checkered homespun wool with a solid-colored inset. The hem is bordered by a broad strip of red woolen fabric and trimmed with narrow strips of tinsel and yellow and blue ribbons.
Inv. No. 96314 B-2257.
159. APRON Homespun linen with a small checkered pattern. Decorated with strips of red calico, blue and yellow ribbon, and pieces of cotton.
Inv. No. 56504 B-1042. Acquired in 1925.
Historical Museum

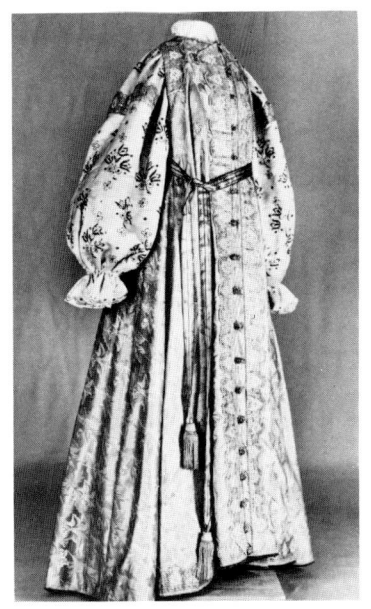

142, 143, 144

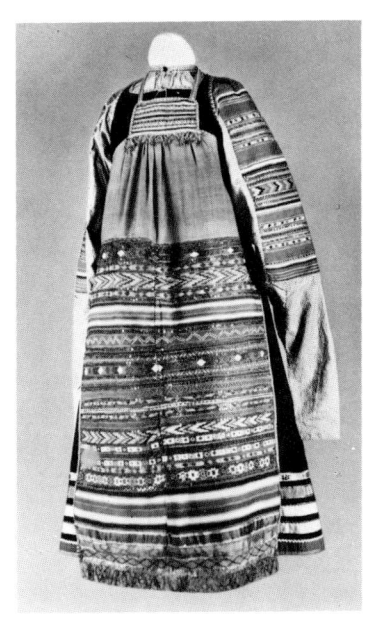

148, 149, 150

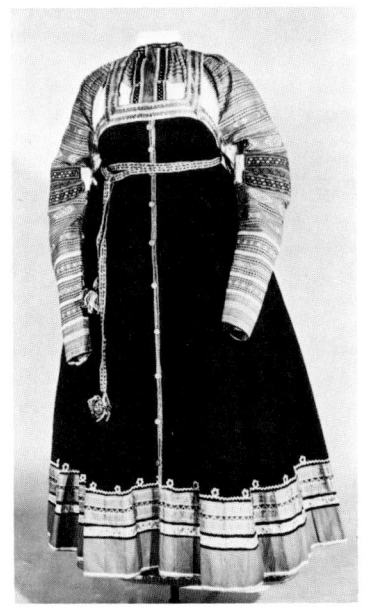

151, 152, 153

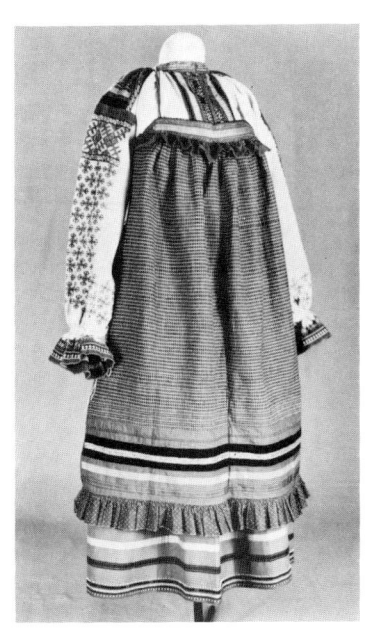

157, 158, 159

Female Peasant's Holiday Dress
Second half of the 19th century. Ryazan region.
160. RUBAKHA Homespun linen canvas. Short, with wide sleeves gathered at the wrist to form a frill. Decorated with strips of red factory-made fabric and embroidery.
Inv. No. 81134 a, B-904. Acquired in 1943.
161. PONEVA (skirt) Blue checkered homespun wool with a solid color cotton insert. Decorated with strips of factory-made fabric, spangles, and white beadwork.
Inv. No. 81134 b B-904. Acquired in 1943.
162. PEREDNIK ZAPON (apron) Linen canvas. Decorated with strips of factory-made fabric and embroidery. The edges are bordered with strips of red calico frills, velvet, embroidered cloth, and handmade lace.
Inv. No. 81134 v B-904. Acquired in 1943.
163. SHUSHPAN (tunic) White homespun wool. Tuniclike, with short sleeves. Decorated with strips of patterned woven cloth, red calico, and cotton. The hem is trimmed with fringe and covered with beadwork.
Inv. No. 55858 B-505. Acquired in 1925.
164. GAITAN (chest ornament) Multicolored beads.
Inv. No. 68862 Ch-107. Acquired in 1930.
165. ROGATAYA KICHKA (headdress) Red calico, gold galloon, and beadwork.
Inv. No. 68862 a, v, g, d, ye-854. Acquired in 1930.
166. BACK ORNAMENT "WINGS" Strips of braided gold, bands, embroidery, and beadwork on a red calico background.
Inv. No. 68862 B-645. Acquired in 1930.
Historical Museum

Female Peasant's Dress
Second half of the 19th century. Kaluga region.
167. RUBAKHA Homespun linen canvas. Full-length. The hem is bordered by narrow strips of red calico, blue cotton, and braiding.
Inv. No. 77859 B/637a. Acquired in 1953.
168. PONEVA (skirt) Checkered homespun wool. Open in front and tied at the waist, like a wraparound. Trimmed with strips of factory-made fabric and galloon.
Inv. No. 87727 B-1663. Acquired in 1953.

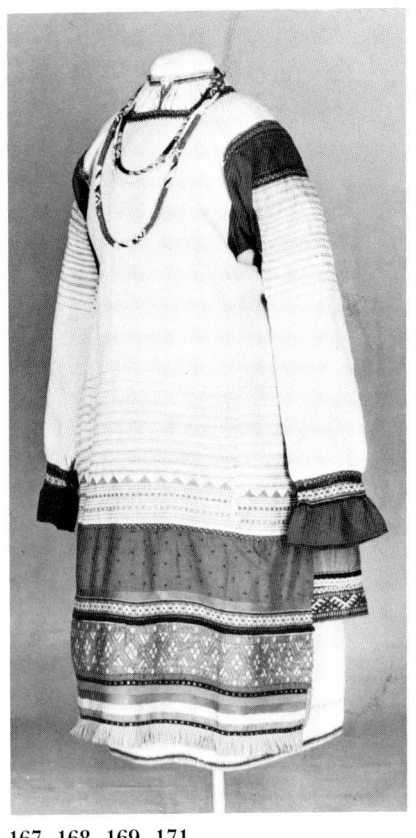
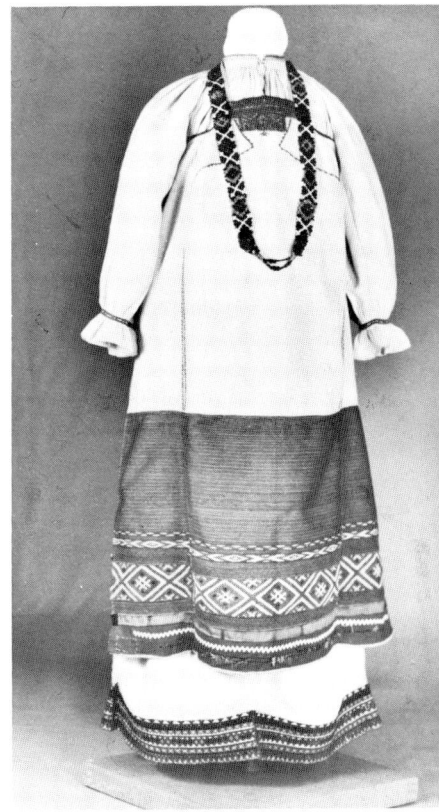

167, 168, 169, 171   172, 173, 174, 176

169. ZAPON (apron) Unbleached linen canvas. With sleeves. Decorated with strips of red calico, embroidery, and ribbons.
   Inv. No. 77859 B/637v. Acquired in 1953.
170. SBORNIK (headdress) Trimmed with swansdown, two strings of beads, and galloon.
   Inv. No. 77859 B/637d. Acquired in 1953.
171. TWO GAITANS Beads.
   Inv. No. 55693 Ch 248, 77859b 637ye. Acquired in 1953.
   Historical Museum

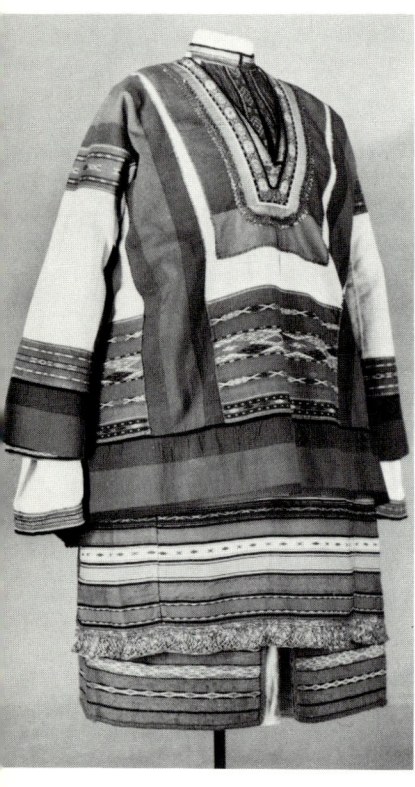 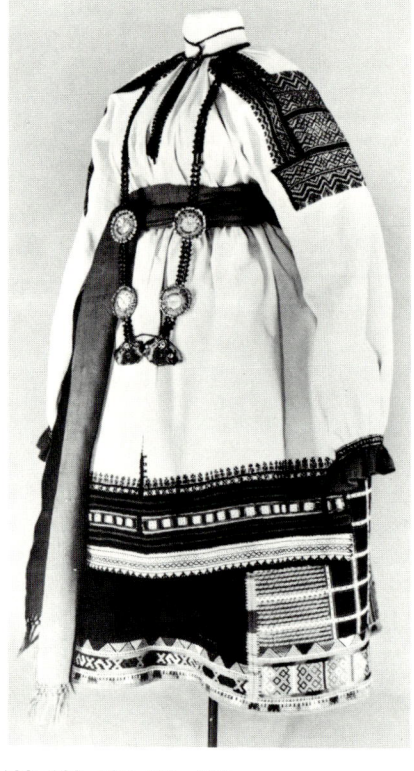

179, 180, 181, 182   188, 189, 190, 191, 192

Female Peasant's Dress
Second half of the 19th century. Orlov region.
172. RUBAKHA Homespun linen canvas. Full-length. The hem is embroidered with wool.
    Inv. No. 95749 V 2130.
173. PONEVA Handwoven wool. Open, trimmed with woolen embroidery and tinsel bone lace.
    Inv. No. 95947/b B2128.
174. APRON Linen canvas. The hem is bordered by a woven pattern and embroidery worked in red thread.
    Inv. No. 95947/59v 2138.

175. HEADDRESS Red calico. The hard front is trimmed with silver galloon and two colorful pompoms at the top.
Inv. No. 95947/10a ye854.
176. GAITAN (chest ornament) Beads.
Inv. No. 16719 Ch-255. Acquired in 1902.
Historical Museum

Maiden's Holiday Dress
Second half of the 19th century. Tula region.
177. RUBAKHA Homespun linen canvas. Long-sleeved with inserts in the underpart of the sleeve. Decorated with strips of red calico, embroidery, and sequins.
Inv. No. 97407 B-2334. Acquired in 1959.
178. BELT TO THE RUBAKHA Homespun red wool, the ends covered in beadwork.
Inv. No. 84107 I-587. Acquired in 1953.
Historical Museum

Female Peasant's Holiday Dress
19th century. Penza region.
179. RUBAKHA Homespun bleached linen. Full-length, with panels cut on the bias. Decorated with a woven pattern in multicolored thread.
Inv. No. 82887 B-1229-2. Acquired in 1949.
180. PONEVA (skirt) Homespun "heavy" wool (warp is hemp). Wrap-around. Decorated with a woven pattern.
Inv. No. 82887 B-1229-1. Acquired in 1949.
181. ZAPON (apron) Homespun linen canvas. Long sleeves. Decorated with a woven pattern.
Inv. No. 82887 B-1230. Acquired in 1949.
182. NAGRUDNIK OUTER GARMENT (sleeved tunic) White thin homespun wool with multicolored bands.
Inv. No. 82887 B-1231. Acquired in 1949.
183. SOROKA (MAGPIE) HEADDRESS Soft, of red cotton, trimmed with strips, spangles, and shells.
Inv. No. 82887 Ye 635. Acquired in 1949.
Historical Museum

Female Peasant's Holiday Dress
Late 19th-early 20th century. Tambov region.
184. RUBAKHA Linen canvas with inserts of patterned calico. Short. Decorated with strips of red calico, embroidery, and sequins.
Inv. No. 78316 B674g. Acquired in 1949.
185. PONEVA (skirt) Black checkered homespun wool, with an insert of solid-colored cloth. Trimmed with a woolen braided band.
Inv. No. 78635/2 B-678. Acquired in 1949.
186. ZAPON (apron) Red factory-made wool. Long, with sleeves. Decorated with a woven pattern, ribbons, sequins, and fringes.
Inv. No. 78635/3 B-678. Acquired in 1949.
187. SHORT OUTER GARMENT (SHUSHPAN) Tuniclike, closed at the neck, decorated with woolen embroidery and strips of woven pattern.
Inv. No. 78316 B-674 ye. Acquired in 1949.
Historical Museum

Female Peasant's Dress
Late 19th century. Voronezh region.
188. RUBAKHA Linen canvas. Short, with long sleeves, cut straight. Decorated with couched black cotton thread.
Inv. No. 92003/10 v 1869. Acquired in 1960.
189. PONEVA (skirt) Checkered homespun wool. Solid color insert. Decorated with embroidery solidly covering the background worked in wool thread. The hem is bordered with a strip of embroidery in a geometric pattern.
Inv. No. 97036/2 B-2269. Acquired in 1960.
190. APRON Linen canvas. Belted at the waist. Decorated with black embroidery, ribbons, and galloon.
Inv. No. 97380/29 B-2410. Acquired in 1960.
191. BELT Green homespun wool.
Inv. No. 84824/43 i579 ye. Acquired in 1960.
192. GAITAN (neck ornament) Black beads with gold medallions.
Inv. No. 97036/B-2296.
Historical Museum

Peasant Girl's Dress
Second half of the 19th century. Orlov region.
193. SARAFAN Red patterned calico. Cut straight, held up by straps.

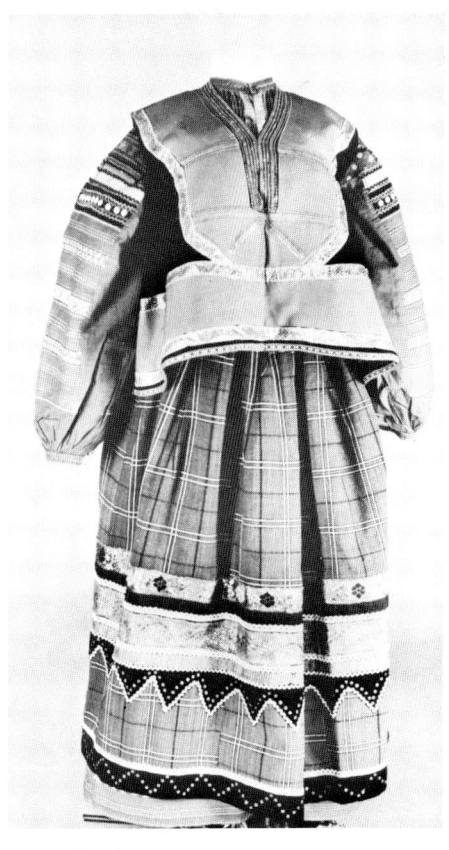 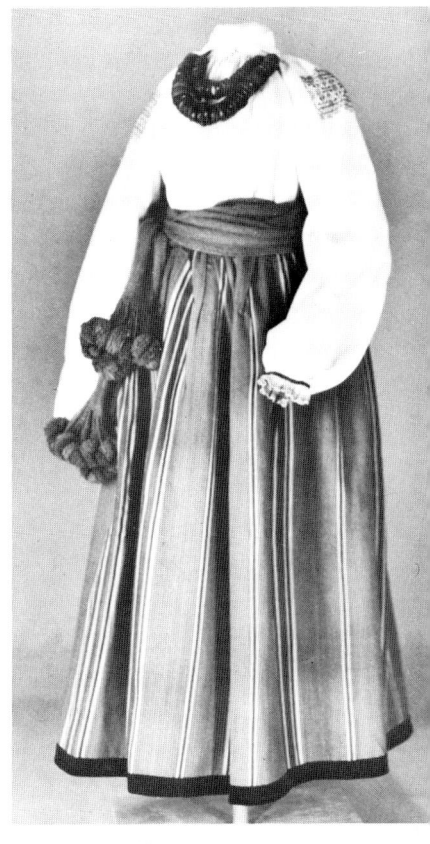

195, 196, 197   201, 202, 203

194. RUBAKHA Cotton with inserts of red cotton. Decorated with metal spangles.
   Inv. No. 96366 B-2272 a, b. Acquired in 1959.
   Historical Museum

Female Peasant's Dress
Late 19th-early 20th century. Ryazan region.
195. RUBAKHA Red patterned calico. Full-length. Sleeves are of woven red patterned cloth. Trimmed with bands and tiny buttons.
   Inv. No. 102706/2 B-3291. Acquired in 1973.

196. PONEVA (skirt) Red checkered homespun wool. No inserts. The hem is bordered by wide strips of red cotton, black cotton velvet, tinsel, and metal spangles.
Inv. No. 99627 B-3292 a. Acquired in 1973.
197. NAGRUDNIK OUTER GARMENT (vest) Black homespun wool. Short, decorated with broad bands of red factory-made wool trimmed with galloon and spangles.
Inv. No. 71032 B-340. Acquired in 1973.
Historical Museum

Female Peasant's Dress
Late 19th century. Kursk.
198. RUBAKHA White cotton. Floral embroidery worked in crossstitch.
Inv. No. 64522 B-473 b.
199. SARAFAN Dark blue homespun wool. Closed at the neck, held up by straps. Pleated skirt. Front of bodice is embroidered in multicolored woolen thread. The hem is bordered by wide strips of factory-made fabric and ribbons.
Inv. No. 52259 B-471.
200. BELT Homespun wool. Fringes at the ends.
Inv. No. 64524 B-473b. Acquired in 1920s.
Historical Museum

Female Peasant's Dress
Second half of the 19th century. Voronezh region.
201. RUBAKHA Patterned bleached linen canvas. Short, with turndown collar. Sleeves embroidered with bands of woven red pattern.
Inv. No. 83840 B-1593. Acquired in 1951.
202. SKIRT Red narrow-striped homespun wool. The hem is paneled with blue cotton velvet.
Inv. No. 102449/27 B-3353. Acquired in 1972.
203. BELT Braided red homespun wool. Red and green tassels at the ends.
Inv. No. 80753 I-451. Acquired in 1940.
204. KOLYASKI NECKLACE Crude amber.
Inv. No. 83487/3 Ch-320. Acquired in 1952.
Historical Museum

Peasant Maiden's Dress
Late 19th century. Kaluga region.
205. RUBAKHA Homespun linen canvas. Full-length, paneled with a woven red pattern and insets of red calico.
Inv. No. 82929 B-1218. Acquired in 1924.
206. APRON Canvas. Short, embroidered in multicolored threads worked in herringbone stitch.
Inv. No. 54784 B-1033. Acquired in 1924.
Historical Museum

Woman's Dress
19th century. Russia.
207. SARAFAN Black silk. Panels cut on the bias, open in front, with twenty metal buttons down the front.
Inv. No. 83269 B-1457. Acquired in 1951.
208. RUBAKHA White cotton.
Inv. No. 80793/2 B-920. Acquired in 1940.
Historical Museum

Male Peasant's Dress
Late 19th century. Arkhangelsk region.
209. RUBAKHA Coarse multicolored homespun linen. Tuniclike, with side panels cut on the bias.
Inv. No. 101275 B-2942. Acquired in 1969.
210. TROUSERS Homespun linen canvas.
Inv. No. 93303/2 B-3301. Acquired in 1963.
211. BELT Gold and black.
Inv. No. 83206 I-2544.
Historical Museum

Male Peasant's Dress
19th century. Penza region.
212. RUBAKHA Homespun linen canvas. Tuniclike, trimmed with embroidery.
Inv. No. 79798 B-691. Acquired in 1938.
213. TROUSERS Homespun linen canvas.
Inv. No. 84107 B-1770/27. Acquired in 1962.
214. BELT Yellow.
Inv. No. 23396 I 235.
Historical Museum

215. **Poddyovka** (woman's long-waisted coat)
Homespun dark brown broadcloth with multicolored braid.
Late 19th century. Voronezh region.
Inv. No. 92003/7 B-1871. Acquired in 1956.
Historical Museum

216. **Shuba** (woman's coat)
Purple brocade with squirrel fur lining and fur collar. Very full sleeves. Late 19th century. Northern Russia.
Inv. No. 96363 Kp 421.
Historical Museum

217. **Rubakha** (man's holiday shirt)
Homespun linen canvas decorated with a woven pattern.
Inv. No. 98301/2 B-2957. Acquired in 1963.
Historical Museum

218. **Rubakha Kosovorotka** (man's holiday blouse with a side fastening)
Red silk. Embroidery worked in cross-stitch.
Inv. No. 96791 B-2299. Acquired in 1960.
Historical Museum

219. **Kartuz** (man's visored cap)
Bast. Novgorod region. 1880s.
Inv. No. 78336 Ye-377. Acquired in 1936.
Historical Museum

220. **Poneva** (skirt)
Homespun checkered wool with an inset. Embroidered in multicolored woolen thread worked in broad chain and buttonhole stitches. Late 19th century. Voronezh region.
Inv. No. 97480/20 B-2406. Acquired in 1961.
Historical Museum

221. **Poneva** (skirt)
Checkered homespun wool with an inset. Decorated with embroidery, spangles, and a woven pattern. Second half of the 19th century. Bryansk.

Inv. No. 18110 B-493. Acquired in 1889.
Historical Museum

222. **Apron**
Bleached homespun linen canvas with embroidered pattern worked in red linen thread. Second half of the 19th century. Vologda region.
Inv. No. 54784 B-1024. Acquired in 1924.
Historical Museum

223. **Navershnik** (children's tuniclike outer garment)
Homespun linen canvas with red bands, drawnwork, and embroidery. Mid-19th century. Smolensk region.
Inv. No. 83005 B-1456. Acquired in 1949.
Historical Museum

224. **Koruna** (maiden's headdress)
Worked in seed pearls, colored glass, and silk ribbon worked in gold thread. Late 18th-early 19th century.
Inv. No. 54787 Kr. B-679. Acquired in 1924.
Historical Museum

225. **Maiden's Headdress**
Pink brocade worked with galloon, mother-of-pearl, and gold spangles. 18th century. Northern Russia.
Inv. No. 17838 Kr. B-641. Acquired in 1889.
Historical Museum

226. **Kokoshnik** (woman's holiday headdress)
Stiff cap, worn toward back of head, rising and widening toward the front. Worked in gold thread, seed pearls, metal spangles, and mother-of-pearl. 18th century. Vologda region.
Inv. No. 15898 Ye-160. Acquired in 1887.
Historical Museum

227. **Kokoshnik**
Gold thread laid in rows and couched down on red velvet background. 18th century. Nizhny Novgorod region.
Inv. No. 77655 Ye-242. Acquired in 1935.
Historical Museum

228. Kokoshnik
Red velvet worked with gold thread and metal spangles. The wide front is trimmed with tinsel, beads, and colored glass. Late 18th-early 19th century.
Inv. No. 78014 Ye-311. Acquired in 1936.
Historical Museum

229. Kokoshnik
Moss green silk embroidered with silver, pearls, mother-of-pearl, and colored stones. Late 18th-early 19th century. Kostroma region.
Inv. No. 77655/155 Ye-495.
Historical Museum

230. Kokoshnik
Red velvet densely embroidered in gold with front fringe of mother-of-pearl. Early 19th century. Tver region.
Inv. No. 33593 90.
Historical Museum

231. Kokoshnik
Red velvet worked in gold thread. The back is trimmed with silk ribbons. Early 19th century.
Inv. No. 54786 Krv 328. Acquired in 1929.
Historical Museum

232. Kokoshnik
Red velvet worked in gold thread and metal spangles. Trimmed with yellow silk ribbon. Late 18th-early 19th century. Moscow region.
Inv. No. 70488 Ye 637. Acquired in 1936.
Historical Museum

233. Kokoshnik
Red velvet worked in gold thread. The high front is paneled with a wide strip of gold galloon. 19th century.
Inv. No. 34048 Kr. 178. Acquired in 1896.
Historical Museum

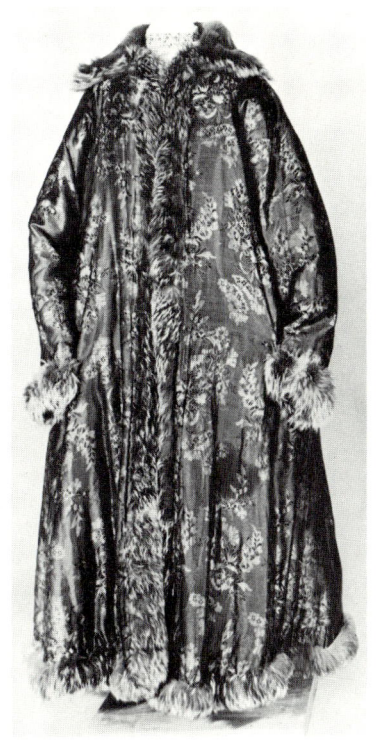

216

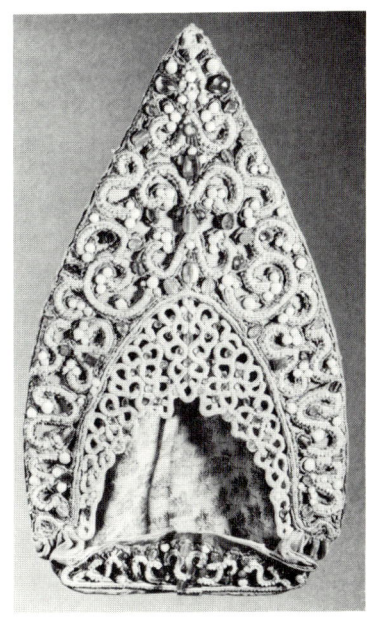

229

227

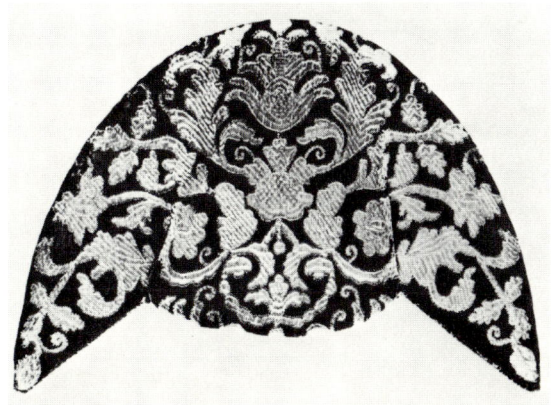

234. **Nakosnik** (woman's hair decoration)
Worked with gold and silver thread laid in rows couched down on red velvet background. Floral design. Triangular. Gold bone lace is sewn to the lower edge. 18th century. Russian work.
Inv. No. 22958 shch Kr. B-690. Acquired in 1905.
Historical Museum

235. **Nakosnik**
The front is of red velvet, the back of brown corded material. Embroidered with gold thread and colored tinsel; the design represents a bird on a twig. Triangular. Decorated with fringes of gold thread. 18th century. Russian work. Size: 9 x 7.5 cm.
Inv. No. 36290 Kr. B-704. Acquired in 1898.
Historical Museum

236. **Nakosnik**
Silk embroidered with gold threads and touches of tinsel. Triangular. Decorated with gold galloon. 18th century. Russian work.
Inv. No. 54788 Kr. B-689. Acquired in 1924.
Historical Museum

237. **Nakosnik**
Gold thread laid in rows and couched down with the same thread. Triangular. Solidly worked in large mother-of-pearl plates and colored glass on gold tinsel background. Early 18th century. Russian work.
Inv. No. 22955 Kr. B-699.
Historical Museum

238. **Nakosnik**
Embroidered with gold and silver threads. Bow-shaped. Second half of the 18th century. Russian work.
Inv. No. 22972 shch 734. Acquired in 1906.
Historical Museum

239. **Earrings** (pair)
Silver gilt set with pearls and mother-of-pearl. First quarter of the 18th century. Russia. Size: 5.8 x 4 cm.
Inv. No. 17389 shch/ok 16067 ZV-3578. Acquired in 1905.
Historical Museum

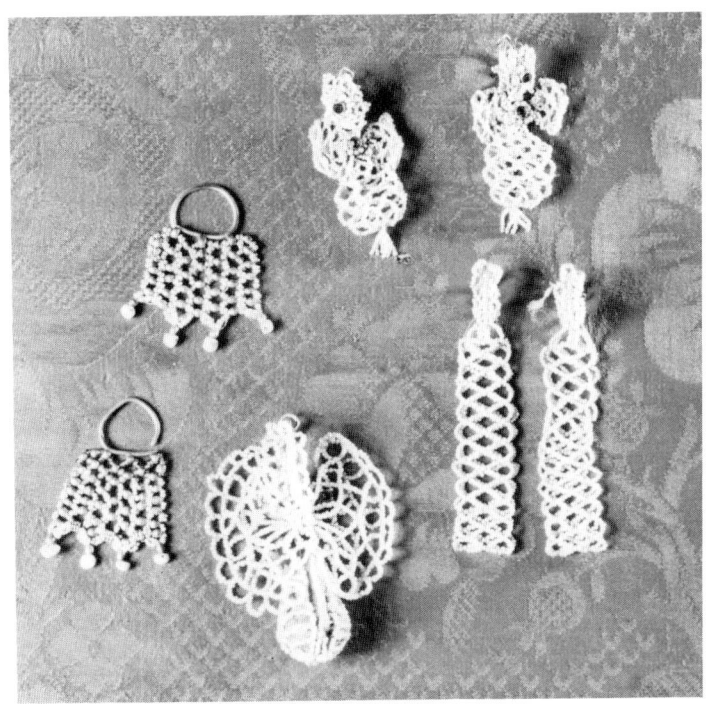

239, 240, 241, 242

240. Earrings (pair)
Silver gilt and copper set with pearls. Lacelike pendants are set with pearls. Mid-18th century. Russia. Size: 9 x 1.8 cm.
   Inv. No. 17391 shch/ok 15095 ZV-3559. Acquired in 1905.
   Historical Museum

241. Earrings (pair)
Low-standard silver set with pearls and glass. Oval bow-shaped pendant earrings with a tassel. Late 18th-early 19th century. Russia. Size: 6.5 x 2.7 cm.
   Inv. No. 55006/ok 15105 ZV-3551. Acquired in 1905.
   Historical Museum

242. Earrings (pair)
Threaded pearls with a pendant in the form of a pear-shaped

design studded with seed pearls. Late 18th-early 19th century. Olonetsk. Size: 7.5 x 6 cm.
Inv. No. 99932/ok 16263 ZV-9862. Acquired in 1966.
Historical Museum

243. **Cross on a Chain**
Solid silver. 18th century. Russia. Cross: 11.3 x 11.3 cm. Length of chain: 82 cm.
Inv. No. 35989/ok 10316 SB-2180. Acquired in 1898.
Historical Museum

244. **Pectoral**
Cut mother-of-pearl and glass set in metal. Early 19th century. Northern Russia.
Inv. No. 35434 Ch-209. Acquired in 1898.
Historical Museum

245. **Button**
Silver gilt. Spherical. Each sphere consists of eight oval petals with two little rings. 18th century. Russia. Size: 2.2 x 1.6 x 1.6 cm.
Inv. No. 19129 shch/ok 21837 SB-9395. Acquired in 1905.
Historical Museum

246. **Button**
Silver gilt. Spherical. Face is decorated with six oval petals and four silver beads. The back of the button is smooth and has a loop for fastening. 18th century. Russia. Size: 3.1 x 2.1 x 2.1 cm.
Inv. No. 53054/ok 22139 SB-9560.
Historical Museum

247. **Button**
Poorly gilded silver. Egg-shaped. Triangular design in smooth setting. 18th century. Russia. Size: 3.3 x 1.8 x 1.7 cm.
Inv. No. 11169 shch/ok 22140 SB-10400. Acquired in 1905.
Historical Museum

248. **Mittens**
Wool decorated with gold embroidery. Late 18th-early 19th century. Russian work.

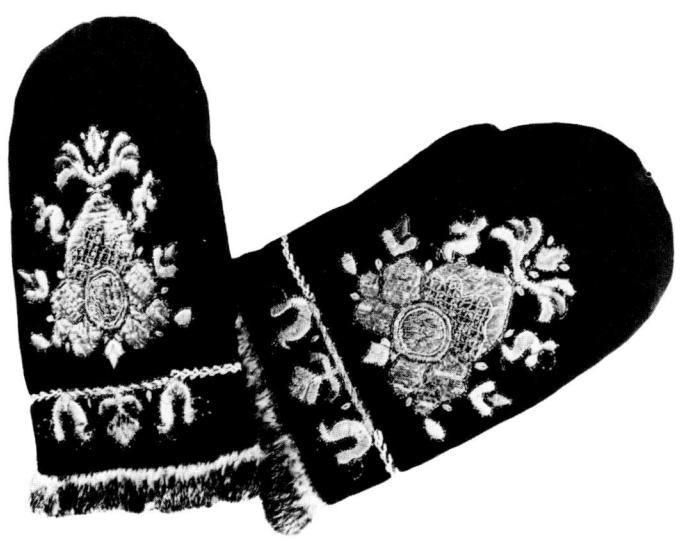

248

Inv. No. 55743a, b R-74. Acquired in 1924.
Historical Museum

249. Mittens
Velvet decorated with gold embroidery. Late 18th-early 19th century. Russian work.
Inv. No. 18359 R-71. Acquired in 1899.
Historical Museum

250. Gloves
Wool decorated with gold embroidery. Late 18th-early 19th century. Russian work.
Inv. No. 57102 R-116 a, b. Acquired in 1925.
Historical Museum

251. Woman's Holiday High Boots
Leather. Gathered at the calf, counter is decorated with metal nails. Layered heels decorated with a horseshoe. Early 20th century. Ryazan.
Inv. No. 80169 Zh-140 a, b. Acquired in 1939.
Historical Museum

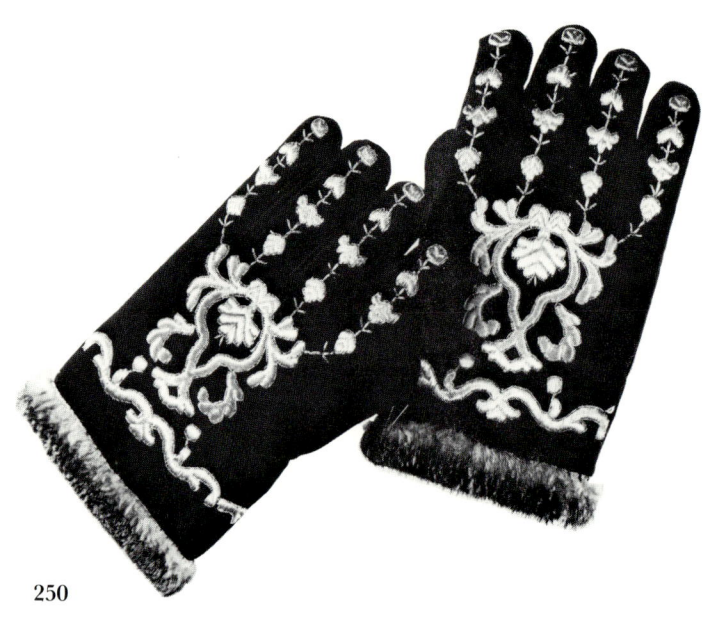

250

252. **Woman's Bast Shoes**
Early 20th century. Smolensk region.
Inv. No. 98052 Zh-535 a, b. Acquired in 1962.
Historical Museum

253. **Woman's Holiday Bast Shoes**
Early 20th century. Ryazan region.
Inv. No. 103553 a, b Kp 1475 a, b. Acquired in 1953.
Historical Museum

254. **Man's Bast Shoes**
Inv. No. 98052 Zh-537 a, b. Acquired in 1962.
Historical Museum

255. **Kerchief**
Crimson silk embroidered with gold thread in a vegetative pattern. Decorated with gold fringe and woven lettering: S.Sh.F.M.G.K.[?]Ye.A.L. Late 18th century. Russian work. Size: 105 x 103 cm.

Inv. No. 80305/12 D-727. Acquired in 1938.
Historical Museum

256. **Kerchief**
Brocade worked in velvet thread. Late 18th-early 19th century. Russian work. Size: 110 x 105 cm.
Inv. No. 57128 D-9. Acquired in 1929.
Historical Museum

257. **Kerchief**
Pink silk woven with gold, silver, and velvet thread in a vegetative pattern. Decorated with gold fringe. First half of the 19th century. Russian work. Size: 109 x 110 cm.
Inv. No. 78014 D-629.
Historical Museum

258. **Kerchief**
Dull green brocade with a floral pattern. Early 19th century. Russian work. Size: 104 x 99 cm.
Inv. No. 87726 D-819. Acquired in 1955.
Historical Museum

259. **Kerchief**
With a bridal veil. First half of the 19th century. Russian work. Size: 209 x 108 cm.
Inv. No. 54722 D-4. Acquired in 1923.
Historical Museum

260. **Shawl**
Wool. Woven Oriental design, paneled with a border. Second half of the 19th century. Russian work. Size: 194 x 189 cm.
Inv. No. 100839 D-1236. Acquired in 1968.
Historical Museum

261. **Kerchief**
Printed wool. Oriental design, trimmed with fringes. Second half of the 19th century. Russian work. Size: 146 x 156 cm.
Inv. No. 96220 D-1066. Acquired in 1959.
Historical Museum

262. **Kerchief**
Wool. Oriental design printed on a gray background. 19th century. Russia. Size: 162 x 162 cm.
Inv. No. 99649 D-1144. Acquired in 1966.
Historical Museum

263. **Kerchief**
Wool. Oriental design printed on a green background. Manufactured at the factory of Ivan Butikov, Moscow. 19th century. Russia. Size: 124 x 121 cm.
Inv. No. 102701/2 KP-1263/2. Acquired in 1973.
Historical Museum

264. **Kerchief**
Patterned silk, black and orange flowers on a blue background; decorated with tassels along the sides. Second half of the 19th century. Russian work.
Inv. No. ERT-17221. Acquired in 1964.
The Hermitage

265. **Kerchief**
Ribbed silk, green and orange on black background; decorated with fringes. Second half of the 19th century. Russian work. Size: 150 x 153 cm.
Inv. No. 100005/3 D-1251. Acquired in 1966.
Historical Museum

266. **Kerchief**
Golden yellow silk with a woven floral pattern. Late 19th century. Russian work. Size: 104 x 102 cm.
Inv. No. 78336/157 D-747. Acquired in 1936.
Historical Museum

267. **Kerchief**
Silk and cotton. Woven floral pattern on a brown background. Second half of the 19th century. Russian work.
Inv. No. 101926 D-1274. Acquired in 1970.
Historical Museum

268. **Kerchief**
Printed red cotton fabric decorated with multicolored fringes. Second half of the 19th century. Russian work. Size: 130 x 111 cm.
Inv. No. 96556/3 D-1053. Acquired in 1959.
Historical Museum

269. **Kerchief**
Red printed with floral pattern. Second half of the 19th century. Russian work. Size: 116 x 115 cm.
Inv. No. 66885 D-238. Acquired in 1929.
Historical Museum

270. **Kerchief**
Red print cotton decorated with fringes. Second half of the 19th century. Russian work. Size: 120 x 108 cm.
Inv. No. 96653/5 D-1069. Acquired in 1959.
Historical Museum

271. **Kerchief**
Cashmere. Printed design on a black ground. Bordered on all edges. Early 19th century. Russian work. Size: 148 x 158 cm. (without the fringe).
Inv. No. 95300/164 D-1017. Acquired in 1957.
Historical Museum

272. **Kerchief**
Wool. Printed floral pattern on a yellow background. Decorated with fringes along the edges. Early 20th century. Moscow region, Pavlov Posad. Size: 154 x 153 cm.
Inv. No. GIM-82807 D-833. Acquired in 1974.
Historical Museum

273. **Kerchief**
Woven red pattern on white ground. Late 19th century. Bryansk.
Inv. No. 103171 Kp-1385/10.
Historical Museum

274. **Kerchief**
Woven red pattern on a white ground. Late 19th century. Bryansk.
Inv. No. 103171 Kp-1385/6.
Historical Museum

275. **Kosynka** (triangular scarf)
Woven red and white fabric with red embroidery. Bordered with a cotton frill. Second half of the 19th century. Northern Russia.
Inv. No. 77645/3 B-475. Acquired in 1935.
Historical Museum

276. **Kerchief**
Blue taffeta embroidered with vegetative design worked in gold and silver threads. Decorated with fringes. Late 18th-early 19th century. Russian work.
Inv. No. 53977 D-63. Acquired in 1953.
Historical Museum

277. **Kerchief**
Muslin embroidered with vegetative design worked in gold and silver threads. Decorated with fringe of gold threads. Late 18th-early 19th century. Nizhny Novgorod.
Inv. No. 84197 b-1675. Acquired in 1953.
Historical Museum

278. **Bridal Veil**
White tulle. Vegetative design worked in white embroidery. Gold galloon. Mid-19th century. Russian work. Size: 214 x 124 cm.
Inv. No. GIM-47373 D-578. Acquired in 1911.
Historical Museum

Urban Costume from the 18th to the Early 20th Century

Man's Everyday Dress
279. COAT Blue broadcloth. Turndown collar and horizontally slit pockets with fancy flaps. The skirt is arranged in groups of pleats. Buttons and buttonholes are trimmed with silk.
    Inv. No. E/rt-8409. Acquired in 1941.
280. WAISTCOAT Red broadcloth. Buttons and buttonholes trimmed with silver thread. Decorated with silver galloon. Belonged to Peter I. Russian work.
    Inv. No. E/rt-8452. Acquired in 1941.
281. KNEE BREECHES Red broadcloth. Buttons and buttonholes trimmed with silver thread.
    Inv. No. E/rt-8470. Acquired in 1941.
    The Hermitage

Man's Full Dress
282. COAT Red broadcloth decorated with silver embroidery.
    Inv. No. E/rt-8571. Acquired in 1941.
283. WAISTCOAT Unbleached linen trimmed with embroidery worked in silver thread and spun gold. Belonged to Peter I. 1710–1720.
    Inv. No. E/rt-8280. Acquired in 1941.
284. KNEE BREECHES Red broadcloth decorated with silver embroidery.
    Inv. No. E/rt-8440. Acquired in 1941.
    The Hermitage

Man's Full Dress
285. COAT Blue corded material trimmed in silver bone lace and buttons.
    Inv. No. E/rt-8369. Acquired in 1941.
286. WAISTCOAT White and blue patterned silk in vegetative design. Buttons and buttonholes decorated with silver embroidery. Belonged to Peter I. 1710–1720s.
    Inv. No. E/rt-8534. Acquired in 1941.

77

287. KNEE BREECHES Blue corded material trimmed with silver bone lace.
   Inv. No. E/rt-8370. Acquired in 1941.
   The Hermitage

Full-Dress Uniform of the Preobrazhensky Regiment
Believed worn by Peter I at the battle of Poltava. Dated before 1709. Russian work.

288. COAT Green broadcloth with red cuffs and copper gilt buttons.
   Inv. No. E/rt-16753. Acquired in 1941.
289. OFFICER'S NECK SIGN OF DISTINCTION (gorget) Part of the full-dress uniform.
   Inv. No. E/rt-16755. Acquired in 1941.
290. OFFICER'S SCARF Part of the full-dress uniform. Netted silver, blue, red, and gold threads; finished with tassels.
   Inv. No. E/rt-16756. Acquired in 1941.
291. TRICORNERED HAT Part of the full-dress uniform. Black felt.
   Inv. No. E/rt-16754. Acquired in 1941.
   The Hermitage

292. **Dressing Gown**
   Green silk with a vegetative design.' Belonged to Peter I. First quarter of the 18th century.
   Inv. No. E/rt-8550. Acquired in 1941.
   The Hermitage

293. **Jackboots**
   Leather. Thigh-high, thick-heeled, thick-soled, square-toed, with wide tops. Belonged to Peter I. First quarter of the 18th century. St. Petersburg.
   Inv. No. OP 143 okhr. 150.
   Kremlin Museums

294. **Wedding Gown** (bodice, skirt, and train)
   Silver brocade embroidered with silver thread and spun gold. Belonged to Grand Princess Catherine (Catherine II). 1745. Russia (?).
   Inv. No. OP 156 okhr. 168.
   Kremlin Museums

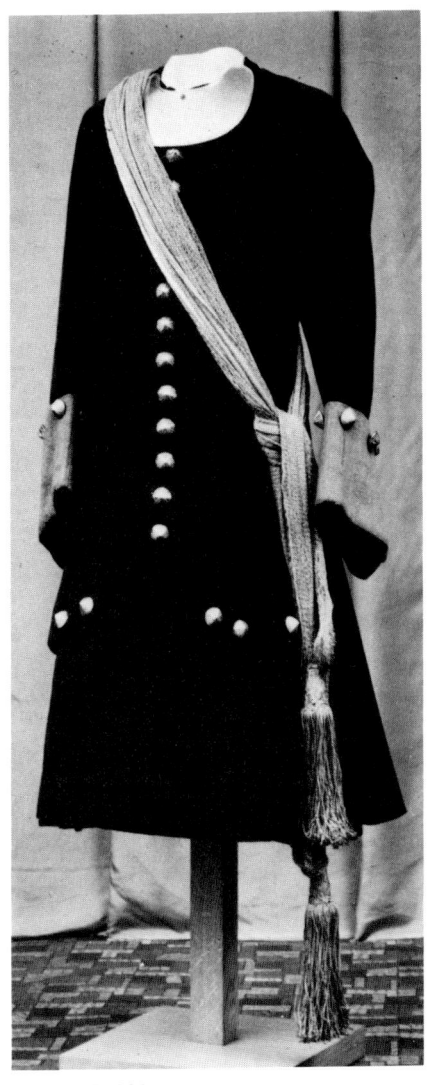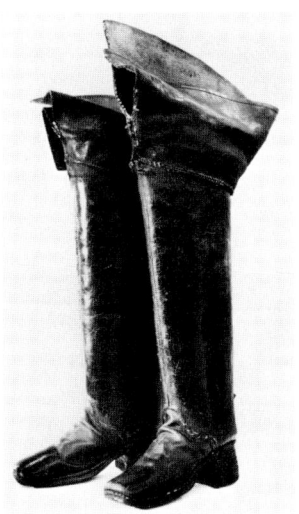

288, 289, 290   293

295. Gown
Brick red silk. "Watteau" back with train falling in ample folds to the ground. Square decolletage and sleeves that are narrow at the shoulder and open out to a rich flounce. Trimmed with falbala.
Inv. No. E/rt-16017. Acquired in 1923.
296. PETTICOAT Pink quilted silk satin. Mid-18th century.
Inv. No. E/rt-14964. Acquired in 1923.
The Hermitage

Man's Full Dress
297. COAT Green broadcloth decorated with gold embroidery. Buttons are covered with cloth. 1727–1730. France.
Inv. No. 232 okhr. 213 op.
298. WAISTCOAT Green broadcloth decorated with gold embroidery. Buttons are covered with cloth. Coat and waistcoat belonged to Emperor Peter II. 1727–1730. France.
Inv. No. 233 okhr. 213 op.
Kremlin Museums

299. **Full-Dress Uniform of the Equestrian Regiment of the Life Guards**
Blue silk. Open in front. With a train and wide pendant sleeves. Worn over a red silk, high-necked, long-sleeved dress. Ornamented with uniform gold galloon and buttons. Belonged to Empress Catherine II. 1770. Russian work.
Inv. Nos. E/rt-11002, 11008. Acquired in 1941.
300. STAR OF THE ORDER OF ST. ANDREW PROTOKLETOS Needlework. Second half of the 18th century.
Inv. No. IO-1383
The Hermitage

301. **Full-Dress Uniform of the Infantry Regiment of the Guards**
Green silk ornamented with gold uniform galloon and buttons. With matching petticoat. Belonged to Catherine II. 1763. Russia.
Inv. Nos. E/rt-11014, 11023. Acquired in 1941.
The Hermitage

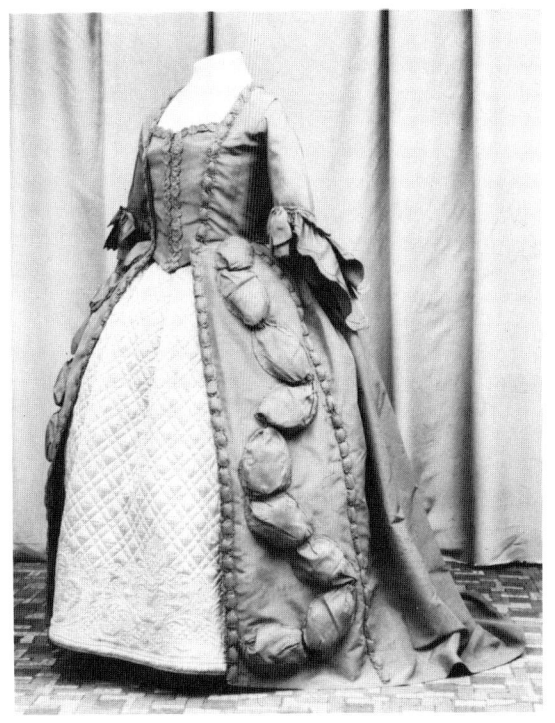

295

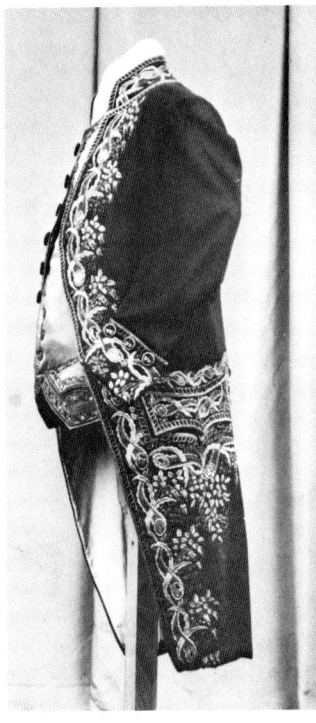

318, 319

302. **Full-Dress Naval Uniform**
 White silk. Open in front with a train and pendant sleeves. Worn over a dress of green silk, with back and sleeves of white silk; trimmed with gold embroidery and copper gilt buttons. Belonged to Catherine II. 1770. Russian work.
 Inv. Nos. TsKh-2687, 2688-P. Acquired in 1946.
 Pavlovsk Museum

Full-Dress Uniform of an Officer of the Equestrian Regiment of the Life Guards

303. COAT Blue broadcloth with scarlet collar and cuffs.
 Inv. No. E/rt-11034. Acquired in 1941.
304. WAISTCOAT Scarlet silk with gold galloon and gold buttons.
 Inv. No. E/rt-11035. Acquired in 1941.

81

305. BREECHES Scarlet broadcloth. Mid-18th century. Russian work.
Inv. No. E/rt-11053. Acquired in 1941.
The Hermitage

Woman's Full Dress
306. DRESS Brown and coral striped silk. Bodice front and petticoat of white satin striped silk. Embroidered with colored silk worked in satin stitch and accented with spangles. Dress is low-necked with elbow-length sleeves and train; open in front. 1780s.
Inv. No. E/rt-8584 a, b. Acquired in 1941.
307. SHOES Light-colored silk. Pointed and moderately high-heeled. Trimmed with embroidery worked in metallic thread and colored glass. Second half of the 18th century.
Inv. No. E/rt-2549 a, b. Acquired in 1941.
The Hermitage

308. Woman's Full Dress
Bodice and train of embossed striped coral velvet. Skirt of silver brocade. Decorated with embroidery worked in colored silk, gold thread, and tiny gilt plates. Belonged to Grand Princess Catherine Pavlovna. 1780.
Inv. Nos. TsKh-2752, 2753, 2754-P.
Pavlovsk Museum

Man's Full Dress
309. COAT Black and white patterned silk. Standing collar, with front sharply cut back on the bias, trimmed with colored embroidery worked in satin stitch with a vegetative design.
Inv. No. E/rt-15573. Acquired in 1941.
310. WAISTCOAT White silk with embroidery similar to that of the coat. 1780s.
Inv. No. E/rt-15574. Acquired in 1941.
311. KNEE BREECHES Black and white patterned silk.
Inv. No. E/rt-15575. Acquired in 1941.
The Hermitage

Boy's Full Dress
312. COAT Pink satin woven with silver pin dots.
Inv. No. E/rt-15578. Acquired in 1941.

313. WAISTCOAT White silk satin trimmed with embroidery worked in gold and silver thread, spun gold, and spangles. 1784.
Inv. No. E/rt-15579. Acquired in 1941.
314. KNEE BREECHES Pink satin woven with silver pin dots.
Inv. No. E/rt-15579. Acquired in 1941.
The Hermitage

Boy's Full Dress
315. COAT Coral velvet.
Inv. No. E/rt-15988. Acquired in 1941.
316. WAISTCOAT Silver brocade trimmed with embroidery worked in gold thread, spun gold, and spangles. 1784.
Inv. No. E/rt-15989. Acquired in 1941.
317. KNEE BREECHES Coral velvet.
Inv. No. E/rt-15989. Acquired in 1941.
The Hermitage

318. **Coat**
Green broadcloth. High standing collar, cuffed long narrow sleeves, figured flap pockets, and front cut on the bias. Trimmed with gold and silver thread embroidery in rich vegetative design. Russian work.
Inv. No. E/rt-16010. Acquired in 1923.
The Hermitage

319. **Waistcoat**
Ocher satin worked in metallic embroidery. Late 18th century.
Inv. No. 12717. Acquired in 1941.
The Hermitage

320. **Redingote** (man's coat)
Red velvet lined with white plush; double-breasted with collar. Trimmed with embroidery worked in gold cord and little metallic plates.
Inv. No. E/rt-15568. Acquired in 1941.
The Hermitage

321. **Dress**
White gauze. Low-necked, high-waisted, short-sleeved, with train. Trimmed with embroidery worked in silk, velvet, gold

thread, and sequins. Gold tinsel belt. Late 18th century.
Inv. No. 66062 B-297. Acquired in 1921.
Historical Museum

322. **Full-Dress Uniform of the General-in-Chief**
Green broadcloth with cuffs and turndown collar of red broadcloth. Uniform gold embroidery with an ornament of sprawling laurel leaves. Adorned with smooth gold buttons.
Inv. No. E/rt-16055. Acquired in 1941.
323. WAISTCOAT Red broadcloth with the same embroidery and buttons as the uniform. Uniform and waistcoat belonged to the great 18th-century Russian general, A. V. Suvorov. Late 18th century. Russian work.
Inv. No. E/rt-16056. Acquired in 1941.
The Hermitage

324. **Dress**
White lawn gauze. Low-necked, short-sleeved, high-waisted, with train. Trimmed with cross-stitch white work and drawnwork. 1800s.
Inv. No. 53135 B-53. Acquired in 1922.
Historical Museum

325. **Dress**
White lawn gauze trimmed with embroidery. Low-necked, high-waisted, short-sleeved, with train. Believed to have belonged to A.V. Suvorov's daughter. About 1800.
Inv. No. E/rt-7507. Acquired in 1941.
326. SASH White satin ribbon.
Inv. No. E/rt-7346.
The Hermitage

Woman's Costume
327. DRESS White lawn. Low-necked, high-waisted, sleeveless, with train. Satin stitch embroidery worked in colored threads with tulle insets. 1800s.
Inv. No. E/rt-8660. Acquired in 1941.
328. RIBBON SASH
Inv. No. E/rt-7355

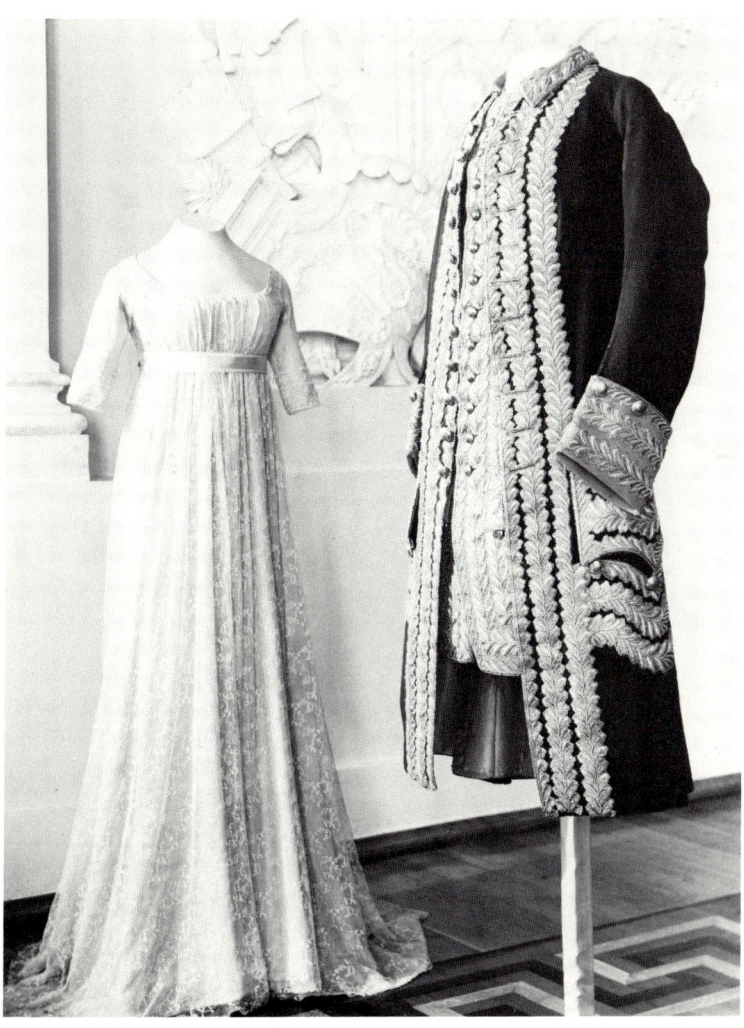

322, 325

329. SHOES Black patterned silk. Flat with pointed toe. 1800s.
Inv. No. E/rt-2532 a, b. Acquired in 1941.
The Hermitage

330. Man's Frock Coat
Red broadcloth. Double-breasted, with collar.
Inv. No. E/rt-11423. Acquired in 1941.

331. VEST Striped silk. Early 19th century.
Inv. No. E/rt-12722. Acquired in 1941.
The Hermitage

Woman's Costume
332. DRESS Pale yellow cashmere. Low-necked, high-waisted, with double sleeves: the outer are short balloon sleeves characteristic of the period, those underneath are long and tight. The bodice, puffed sleeves, and flounces are trimmed with satin stitch embroidery in purple silk along the edges. Late 1810s.
Inv. No. E/rt-8591. Acquired in 1941.
333. SHOES Purple satin and tulle. Square-toed and ornamented with lace, bows, and mother-of-pearl buckles. From the workshop of L. Okler, St. Petersburg. First quarter of the 19th century.
Inv. No. E/rt-2501 a, b.
334. KOLOKOLTSOVSKY SCARF Red wool richly ornamented with a woven floral design. Executed by serf craftsmen. First quarter of the 19th century. Size: 54 x 252 cm.
Inv. No. E/rt-7066. Acquired in 1949.
The Hermitage

Woman's Costume
335. DRESS Crimson silk. High-waisted, high-necked, with collar and long sleeves with epaulets. 1810s.
Inv. No. E/rt-8589. Acquired in 1941.
336. SCARF Brussels lace with a superimposed ornament over tulle. First half of the 19th century.
Inv. No. E/rt-17100. Acquired in 1964.
337. SHOES Red silk embroidered with a tiny floral design. Squaretoed. First quarter of the 19th century.
Inv. No. E/rt-2531 a, b. Acquired in 1941.
The Hermitage

Woman's Summer Street Dress
338. REDINGOTE (lightweight summer coat) Cotton. High-necked, long-sleeved, with a turndown collar and cape. Trimmed with satin stitch and drawn thread white work. Executed by serf craftsmen. 1810s.
Inv. No. E/rt-16835. Acquired in 1960.

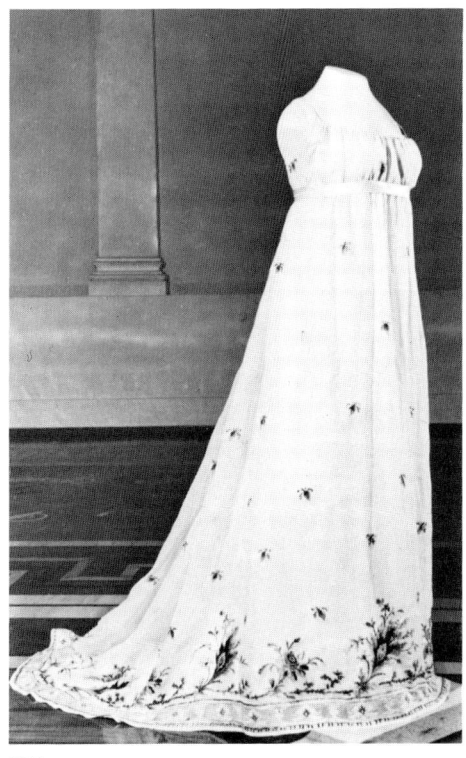

327

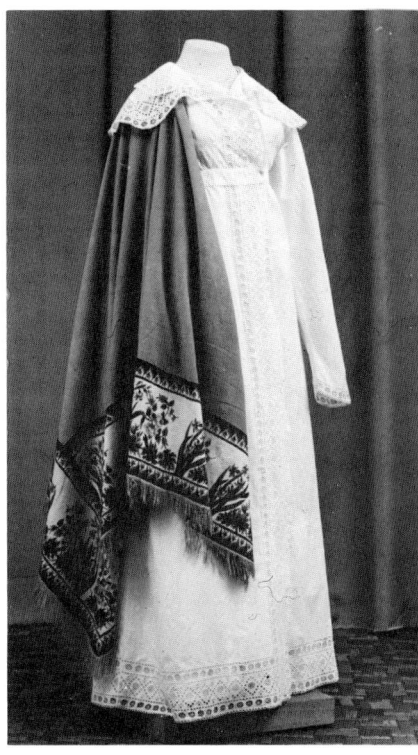

338, 339

339. KOLOKOLTSEVSKAYA SHAWL Blue wool. Borders of floral ornament on white background. Executed by serf craftsmen. First quarter of the 19th century. Russia.
Inv. No. E/rt-7062.
The Hermitage

Woman's Costume

340. DRESS Pink cashmere. Low-necked, high-waisted, with long sleeves puffed at the shoulder. Trimmed with satin cord matching the color of the dress. 1820s.
Inv. No. E/rt-8585 a, b. Acquired in 1941.

341. SCARF Linen bobbin lace. First half of the 19th century. Russian work.
Inv. No. E/rt-16563. Acquired in 1956.
The Hermitage

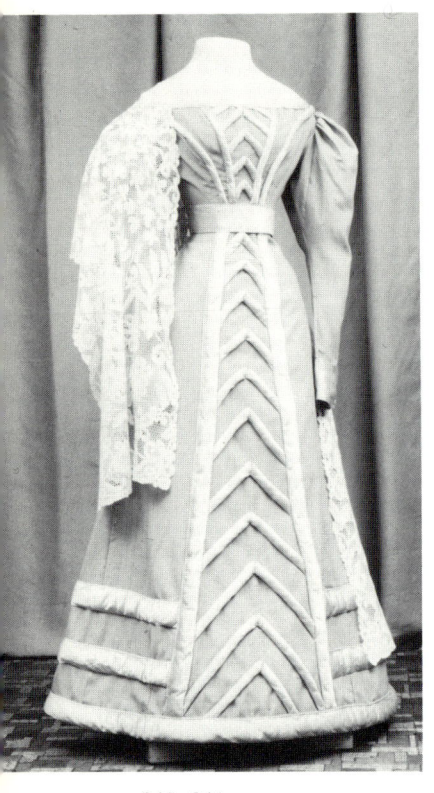 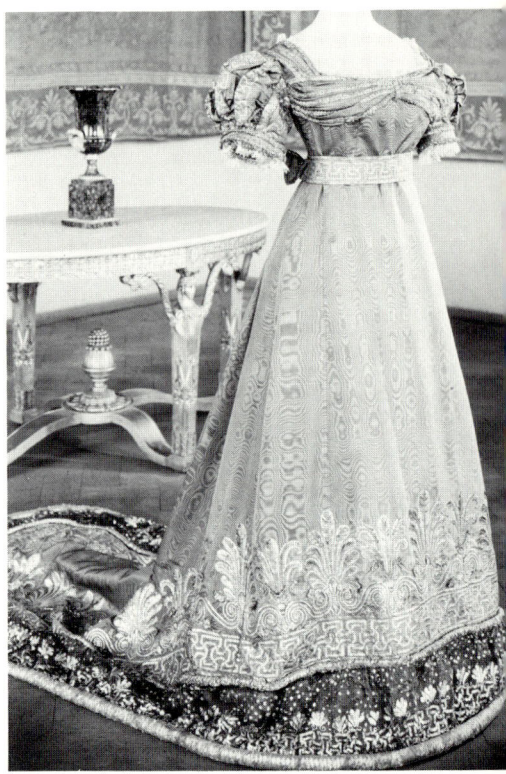

340, 341   342

Woman's Full-Dress

342. DRESS Blue moiré. Low-necked, high-waisted, with short balloon sleeves and train. Bodice, sleeves, and hem trimmed with embroidery worked in gold thread with an elaborate design of broken lines and volutes and an ornament or ancient origin, consisting of radiating petals that spring from a base suggestive of a calyx, that is closely related to the Egyptian lotus and Greek anthemion. 1820s.

    Inv. No. E/rt-8592. Acquired in 1941.

343. HALF BOOTS Gold brocade. Side lacing. First quarter of the 19th century.

    Inv. No. E/rt-2484 a, b. Acquired in 1941.

    The Hermitage

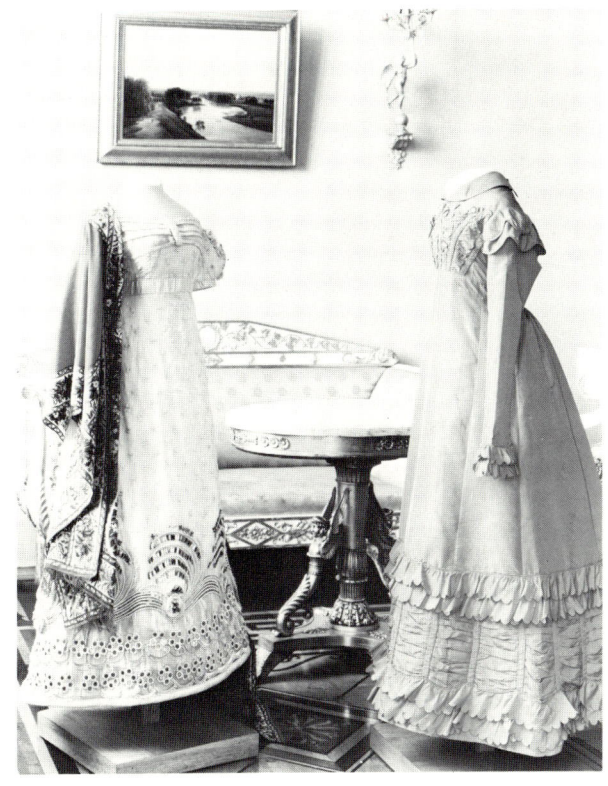

335, 344

344. Ball Dress
White silk tulle. Low-necked, high-waisted, with balloon sleeves. Trimmed with white satin cord and embroidered with metallic thread. 1820s.
   Inv. No. E/rm-8583. Acquired in 1941.
   The Hermitage

345. Dress
White translucent patterned fabric imitative of lace. Low-necked, belted, and trimmed with pink bows. 1830s.
   Inv. No. E/rt-8599 a, b. Acquired in 1941.

346. BELT Steel wire with an oval buckle of polished steel adorned with cut glass in filigree settings. Executed by Tula craftsmen. First half of the 19th century.
Inv. No. E/rt-4896. Acquired in 1941.
The Hermitage

Woman's Dressy Costume
347. DRESS (bodice and skirt) Pale cream faille. Low-necked, sleeveless, with a corsage with folds. Decorated with straw thread embroidery in a vegetative design. 1840s.
Inv. No. E/rt-9483 a, b. Acquired in 1941.
348. CAPE Tulle. Long ends and turndown collar. Trimmed with embroidery and gauze appliqué on tulle. 1840s. Russian work.
Inv. No. E/rt-13976. Acquired in 1941.
The Hermitage

Full-Dress Coat of a Senior Officer of the Hussar Regiment of the Leib Guards
349. DOLOMAN (uniform dress) Crimson broadcloth trimmed with gold cord.
Inv. No. E/rt-11165. Acquired in 1941.
350. MENTIK (short jacket) Crimson broadcloth trimmed with gold cord and rows of buttons. The *mentik* is worn over the *doloman*.
Inv. No. E/rt-11170. Acquired in 1941.
351. PANTALOONS Blue broadcloth decorated with gold galloon.
Inv. No. E/rt-11287. Acquired in 1941.
352. KIVER (headgear) Red wool and black leather with visor.
Inv. No. E/rt-10923 a, b. Acquired in 1941.
353. BOOTS First half of the 19th century.
Inv. No. E/rt-11355 a, b. Acquired in 1941.
354. STAR OF THE ORDER OF ST. GEORGE First half of the 19th century.
Inv. No. IO-1158. Acquired in 1941.
355. RIBBON OF THE ORDER OF ST. GEORGE First half of the 19th century.
Inv. No. E/rt-15254. Acquired in 1941.
The Hermitage
356. SWORD
Inv. No. Z/ZO 302319.
Arsenal Museum

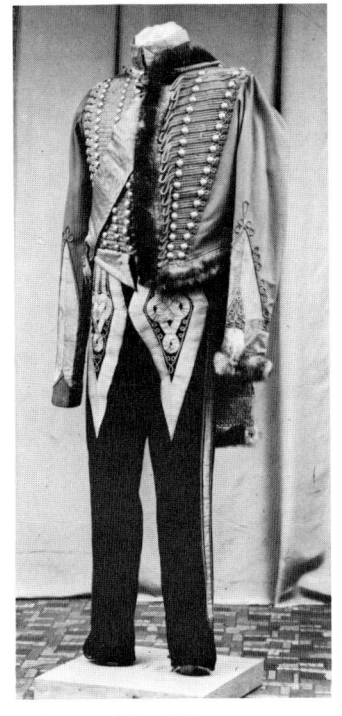 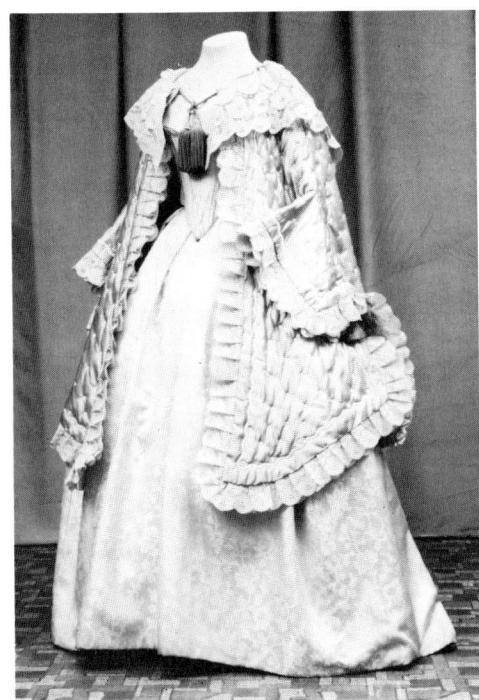

349, 350, 351, 355   357, 358

Woman's Street Dress

357. MANTLE Blue satin and white silk (reversible). Quilted, trimmed with white and blue lace. 1840s. Russian work.
 Inv. No. E/rt-8240. Acquired in 1941.
358. DRESS (bodice and skirt) White patterned silk. Low-necked bodice with folds, short-sleeved. 1840s.
 Inv. No. E/rt-9416 a, b. Acquired in 1941.
 The Hermitage

359. **Dress** (bodice and skirt)
 White lace. Low-necked corsage with folds, short-sleeved, full-skirted, and worn over a white silk satin underdress. 1840s.
 Inv. No. 59065 B-369. Acquired in 1927.
 Historical Museum

360. Dress (bodice and skirt)
Sheer white cotton. High-necked with long sleeves widening at the wrist, tightly fitted bodice, and full skirt with three flounces. Embroidered in purple and white silk and trimmed with ribbons and bows. 1850s.
Inv. No. E/rt-8587 a, b. Acquired in 1941.
The Hermitage

Woman's Costume
361. DRESS Dark green silk satin. High-necked with pagoda sleeves. 1850s.
Inv. No. E/rt-17030. Acquired in 1962.
362. UNDERSLEEVES Lawn with satin stitch embroidery. Mid-19th century. Russian work.
Inv. No. E/rt-8155 a, b. Acquired in 1941.
363. CAPE White silk with appliqué on tulle insets. Fringes. Mid-19th century. Russian work.
Inv. No. E/rt-17683. Acquired in 1970.
364. SHOES Silk satin decorated with embroidery. Low-heeled and square-toed. Mid-19th century.
Inv. No. E/rt-2504 a, b. Acquired in 1941.
The Hermitage

365. Dress
White muslin with multicolored floral print. Pagoda sleeves and high-necked bodice tightly fitted in back and loose and belted in front. Skirt has two flounces bordered with white lace. 1850s.
Inv. No. 57248 B-85. Acquired in 1925.
366. CANZOU White net with embroidery on the collar.
Inv. No. 59370 S-70.
Historical Museum

367. Dress (bodice and skirt)
Green taffeta. High-necked corsage with folds; pagoda sleeves. The skirt consists of two flounces with fringes at the edges. 1850s.
Inv. No. 57249 B-83. Acquired in 1925.
Historical Museum

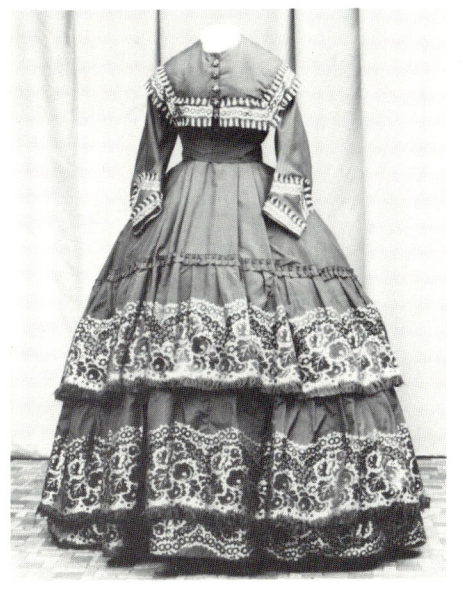

368

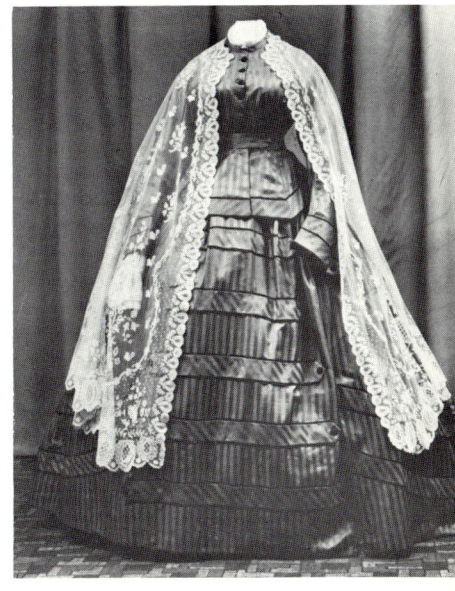

370, 371

368. **Dress**
Blue faille with floral design. High-necked with long sleeves. Trimmed with flounces and fringes. First half of the 1860s.
Inv. No. E/rt-8621. Acquired in 1941.

369. PARASOL Blue silk bordered with floral ornament. 1860s–1870s.
Inv. No. E/rt-6825. Acquired in 1941.
The Hermitage

370. **Dress** (bodice and skirt)
Light brown striped silk. High-necked, tightly fitted bodice, with long sleeves. Second half of the 1860s.
Inv. No. E/rt-12855 a, b. Acquired in 1941.

371. SHAWL White lace.
Inv. No. E/rt-7589.
The Hermitage

372. **Salop** (woman's coat)
Brown silk with blue jacquard vegetative pattern. Quilted, loose, with a cape, round collar, and short sleeves. Trimmed with blue silk fringes along the edges. 1860s.
Inv. No. 84245 B-1706. Acquired in 1954.
Historical Museum

373. **Cape with Hood**
White broadcloth trimmed with tassels and a broad border of satin stitch silk embroidery in a floral pattern. 1860s.
Inv. No. E/rt-17126. Acquired in 1963.
The Hermitage

Woman's Morning Dress
374. PEIGNOIR White lawn. Train and pagoda sleeves. Trimmed with white work and lace. Second half of the 1860s. Russian work.
Inv. No. E/rt-9447. Acquired in 1941.
375. SHOES White lawn with pink lining. High-heeled and square-toed. 1860s.
Inv. No. E/rt-2505 a, b. Acquired in 1941.
The Hermitage

376. **Morning Dress**
White muslin. High-necked, with buttoned-up front fastening and long sleeves. The skirt has a train and is densely gathered at the back and sides. Trimmed with lace and white work. Second half of the 1860s. Russian work.
Inv. No. E/rt-9448. Acquired in 1941.
The Hermitage

377. **Morning Dress**
White patterned cotton. Train. High-necked, tightly fitted bodice, with pagoda sleeves and wide turnback cuffs. Trimmed with satin stitch embroidery and purple silk ribbons. Second half of the 1860s. Russian work.
Inv. No. E/rt-9449. Acquired in 1941.
The Hermitage

378. **Dress of a Woman of the Merchant Class**
Blue-checked taffeta in a geometric design and floral pattern. High-necked, tightly fitted bodice and long sleeves. Trimmed with black machine-made lace. 1860s. Russian work.
Inv. No. E/rt-16721. Acquired in 1958.

379. SHAWL Wool with woven Oriental pattern worked in red, yellow, green, black, and white tones. Second half of the 19th century. Russian manufacture.
Inv. No. E/rt-18401. Acquired in 1974.
The Hermitage

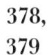
378, 379

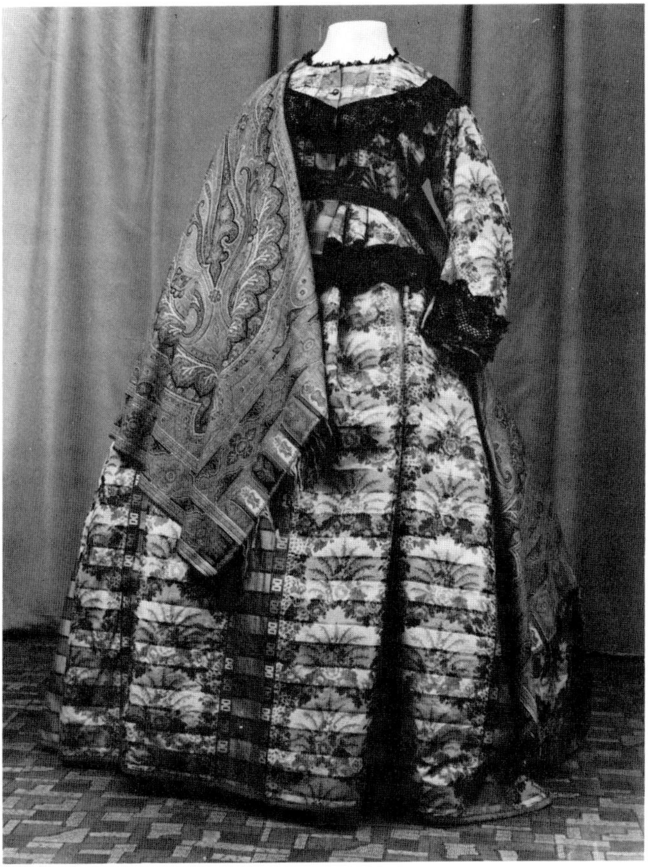

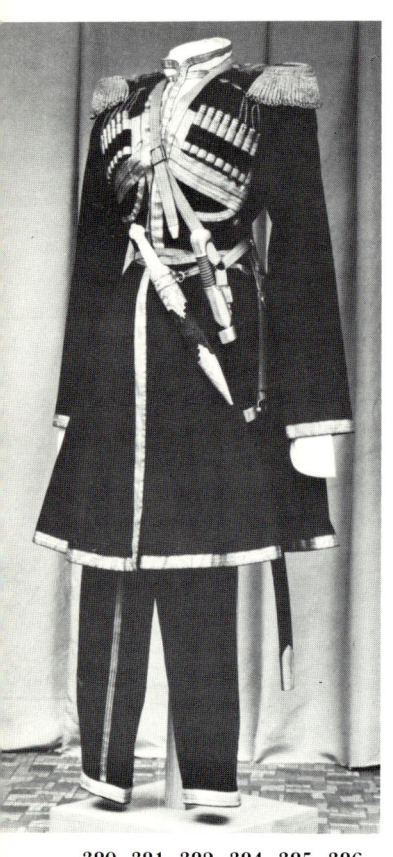 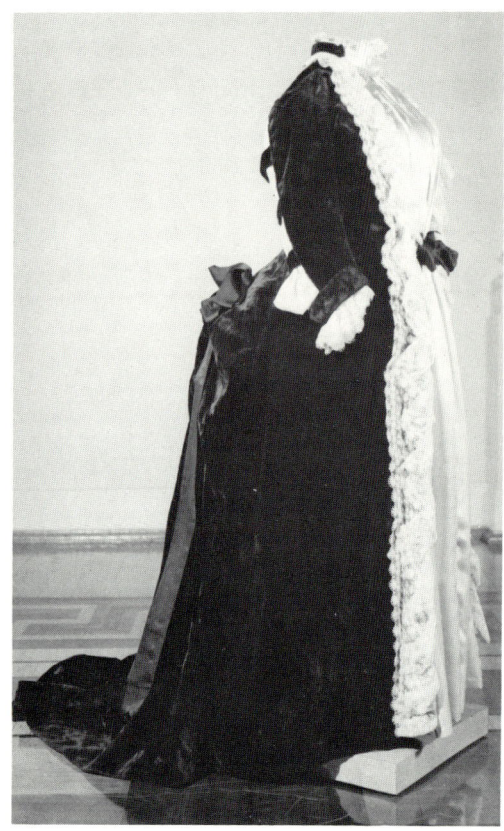

380, 381, 382, 384, 385, 386   387

Uniform of the General of the Cossack Troops

380. CHERKESKA (Circassian long-waisted outer garment) Dark blue broadcloth with silver epaulets. Trimmed with galloon. Fastened to the coat are silver sockets for cartridges, decorated with niello and lined with green velvet.
   Inv. No. E/rt-11315. Acquired in 1941.
381. BESHMET (quilted jacket) White twill trimmed with galloon.
   Inv. No. E/rt-11329. Acquired in 1941.
382. TROUSERS Dark blue broadcloth trimmed with galloon.
   Inv. No. E/rt-11336. Acquired in 1941.

383. PAPAKHA (tall Caucasian hat) Black sheepskin with a top of blue broadcloth. Second half of the 19th century.
Inv. No. E/rt-18138. Acquired in 1972.
384. EPAULETS Silver.
Inv. No. E/rt-10779 SV-1593.
The Hermitage
385. SWORD
Inv. No. Z/ZO 3788.
386. DAGGER
Inv. No. Z/ZO 7684.
Arsenal Museum

Woman's Visiting Costume
387. DRESS Purple velvet. High-necked bodice with standing collar and long sleeves; bustle and train. Trimmed with lavender silk satin, purple ribbons, and lace. 1870s.
Inv. No. E/rt-8649. Acquired in 1941.
388. SHOES White silk satin. Pointed and high-heeled. From I. Yegorov's shoe store, St. Petersburg. 1870s.
Inv. No. E/rt-2485 a, b. Acquired in 1941.
389. HAT White corded silk trimmed with lace and ribbons. Late 1860s–1870s.
Inv. No. E/rt-6108. Acquired in 1941.
390. GLOVES White kidskin trimmed with embroidery. Medium length. 1860s–1870s.
Inv. No. E/rt-6938 a, b. Acquired in 1941.
The Hermitage

391. **Dress**
White moiré. High-necked with bustle, train, and long sleeves. Trimmed with purple silk embroidery and velvet and white lace appliqué. Late 1870s. From the firm of Josephine Brusi, Moscow.
Inv. No. 58324 B-182. Acquired in 1926.
Historical Museum

Woman's Costume
392. DRESS (bodice and skirt) Gray silk. High-necked, tightly fitting bodice; train gathered in puffs. 1880s. Russian work.
Inv. No. E/rt-12905 a, b.

393. MANTLE Black silk trimmed with black beads and a wide black lace flounce. 1880s.
Inv. No. E/rt-8256. Acquired in 1941.
394. HIGH BOOTS Lilac silk. High-heeled with a row of buttons along the side. 1880s.
Inv. No. E/rt-2538 a, b. Acquired in 1941.
The Hermitage

395. **Dress** (bodice and skirt)
White silk satin with multicolored velvet in a floral design. Tightly fitted bodice with small, square decolletage and elbow-length sleeves. Skirt is assymmetrically draped in front and has a train. Richly decorated with tulle, lace, red and green velvet, fringes, and pendants. 1880s. The firm of Worth, Paris.
Inv. No. E/rt-8643, a, b. Acquired in 1941.
The Hermitage

396. **Dress** (bodice, skirt, and train)
Black silk satin. Square decolletage with detachable train and below elbow-length sleeves. Embroidered in black bugle beads and trimmed with lace. Late 1880s–early 1890s. The firm of Worth, Paris.
Inv. No. E/rt-12876 a, b, v. Acquired in 1941.
The Hermitage

Woman's Costume

397. DRESS Beige broadcloth. High-necked with high standing collar and train. Trimmed with chain stitch embroidery and spangles. 1890s. The workshop of N. Lamanova, Moscow.
Inv. No. E/rt-9404. Acquired in 1941.
398. CAPE Beige broadcloth trimmed with openwork. 1890s. The workshop of M. & I. Mandl, Moscow.
Inv. No. E/rt-18129. Acquired in 1972.
The Hermitage

Dress (two bodices and skirt)
399. DAY BODICE Lilac velvet. Tightly fitted with a high standing collar and long, draped sleeves.
Inv. No. E/rt-8622 b. Acquired in 1941.

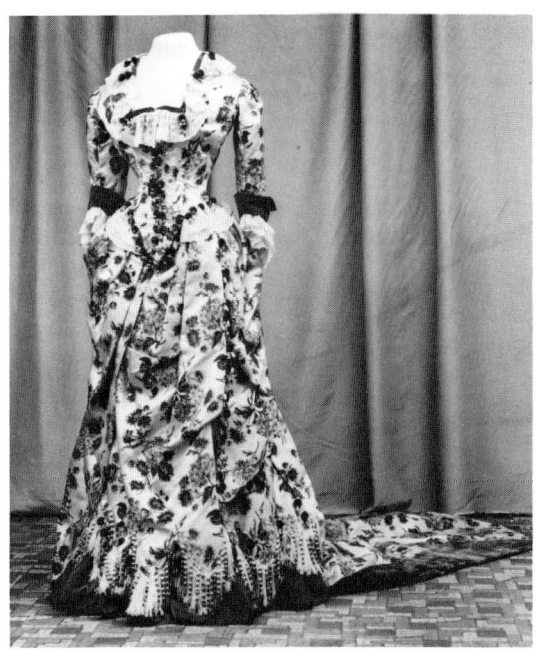

395

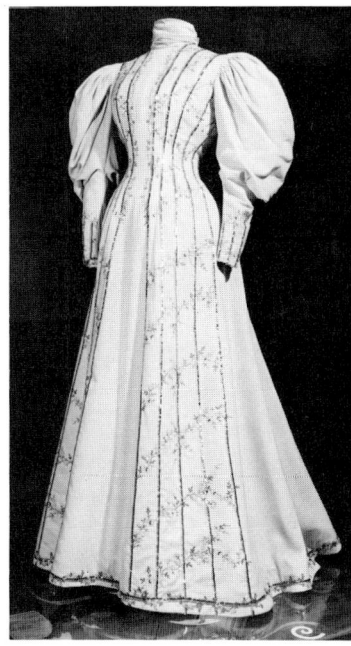

397

400. EVENING BODICE Lilac velvet. Low-necked with elbow-length sleeves; trimmed with lace and embroidered with sequins.
Inv. No. E/rt-8622 v. Acquired in 1941.

401. SKIRT Lilac velvet decorated with a flounce and self cording. The dress is from the firm of Worth, Paris. Second half of the 1890s.
Inv. No. E/rt-8622 a. Acquired in 1941.
The Hermitage

Woman's Full-Dress Court Costume

402. COURT DRESS (bodice, skirt, and train) Silver brocade. Low-necked with pendant sleeves. Detachable train. Trimmed with white marabou and silk embroidery in a vegetative and floral design. Second half of the 19th century. The workshop of Mme. Olga (O. N. Bulbenkova), St. Petersburg.
Inv. No. E/rt-13153 a, b, v. Acquired in 1941.

403. KOKOSHNIK (headdress) Silver brocade with a tulle veil. Richly worked in silver thread. Second half of the 19th century. Russian work.
Inv. No. E/rt-6102, 13139 b. Acquired in 1941.
The Hermitage

Full-Dress Coat of a Gentleman in Attendance
404. UNIFORM Black broadcloth with red collar and cuffs embroidered with gold. Decorated with gilt buttons.
Inv. No. E/rt-10983. Acquired in 1941.
405. TROUSERS White broadcloth with gold stripes.
Inv. No. E/rt-10998. Acquired in 1941.
406. HAT Black felt trimmed with white ostrich plumes and gold embroidery.
Inv. No. E/rt-11537. Acquired in 1941.
407. KEY OF A GENTLEMAN IN ATTENDANCE On a blue ribbon.
Inv. No. E/rt-9627. Acquired in 1941.
408. STAR OF THE ORDER OF ST. VLADIMIR
Inv. No. IO-1160. Acquired in 1941.
409. RIBBON OF THE ORDER OF ST. VLADIMIR
Inv. No. E/rt-9627. Acquired in 1941.
410. SWORD Second half of the 19th century. Russian work.
Inv. No. E/rt-12266 a, b, v. Acquired in 1941.
The Hermitage

Woman's Full-Dress Court Costume
411. COURT DRESS Bodice and train of dark green velvet. White silk satin skirt. Low-necked with pendant sleeves. Trimmed with gold embroidery. Second half of the 19th century. The workshop of Mme. Olga (O. N. Bulbenkova), St. Petersburg.
Inv. No. E/rt-13147 a, b, v. Acquired in 1941.
412. KOKOSHNIK (headdress) Gold brocade worked in imitation pearls, with a tulle veil. Second half of the 19th century. Russian work.
Inv. No. E/rt-6101. Acquired in 1941.
The Hermitage

Formal Full-Dress Coat of a Senator
Second half of the 19th century. Russian work.
413. UNIFORM Red broadcloth with dark green collar and cuffs.

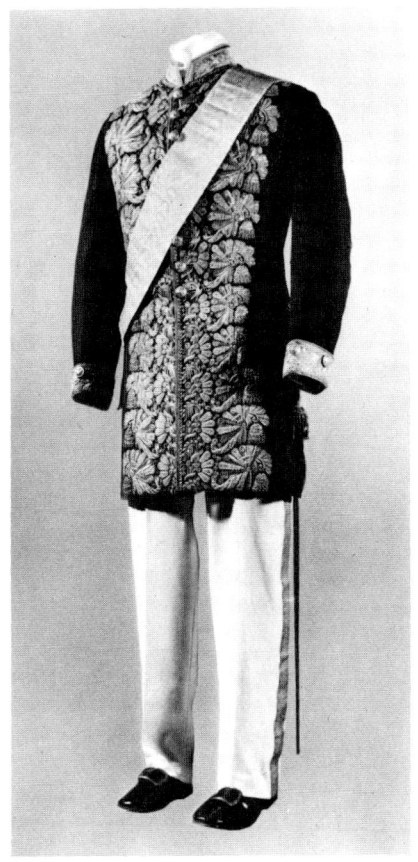

404, 405, 409, 410

Embroidered in an oak and laurel leaf design.
Inv. No. E/rt-10990. Acquired in 1941.
414. TROUSERS White broadcloth with gold stripes.
Inv. No. E/rt-10999. Acquired in 1941.
415. SWORD
Inv. No. E/rt-12258 a, b, v. Acquired in 1941.
416. STAR OF THE ORDER OF ST. ANDREW PROTOKLETOS
Inv. No. E/rt IO-1427. Acquired in 1941.
417. RIBBON OF THE ORDER OF ST. ANDREW PROTOKLETOS
Inv. No. E/rt-9650. Acquired in 1941.
The Hermitage

418. **Court Dress** (bodice, detachable train, cape, and underskirt) Pink silk and white satin trimmed with a vegetative design in silver embroidery. Late 19th–early 20th century. The workshop of N. Lamanova, Moscow.
Inv. No. E/rt-18149 a, b, v. Acquired in 1941.
419. KOKOSHNIK Pink velvet with white lace veil.
Inv. No. 6098.
The Hermitage

Uniform of a Cossack Officer in Attendance
Late 19th–early 20th century. Russian work.
420. CAFTAN-CHEKMEN (outer caftan) With pendant sleeves. Decorated with spun gold frogging, spangles, and galloon. Worn over the *caftan* No. 421.
Inv. No. E/rt-11926. Acquired in 1941.
421. CAFTAN Bright blue broadcloth
Inv. No. E/rt-11923. Acquired in 1941.
422. TROUSERS Black broadcloth trimmed with gold galloon.
Inv. No. E/rt-11915. Acquired in 1941.
423. PAPAKHA (Caucasian hat) Black astrakhan with a blue top. Trimmed with galloon, cord, and a tassel of spun gold.
Inv. No. E/rt-12638. Acquired in 1941.
424. SWORD
Inv. No. E/rt-12251 a, b. Acquired in 1941.
425. BOOTS
Inv. No. E/rt-15402 a, b. Acquired in 1941.
The Hermitage

Full-Dress Uniform of a Blackamoor
Second half of the 19th century. Russian work.
426. SHORT JACKET (undergarment) Dark green broadcloth.
Inv. No. E/rt-11899. Acquired in 1941.
427. SHAROVARY (wide trousers) Red broadcloth trimmed with uniform galloon and gold and silk cord.
Inv. No. E/rt-11904. Acquired in 1941.
428. TWO SLEEVELESS SHIRTS One of white broadcloth, the other of red velvet.
Inv. Nos. E/rt-11946, 11901. Acquired in 1941.
429. FEZ Red broadcloth with a tassel of gold threads.
Inv. No. E/rt-11956. Acquired in 1941.

430. SASH Dark green.
Inv. No. E/rt-11954. Acquired in 1941.

431. LEGGINGS Dark green broadcloth.
Inv. No. E/rt-11962 a, b. Acquired in 1941.

432. SHOES Morocco leather.
Inv. No. E/rt-11970 a, b. Acquired in 1941.
The Hermitage

433. Dressing Gown
Ivory corded silk. High-necked, button-up bodice, ruff collar of cloth and lace, and long sleeves slashed up to the elbow. The bodice is gathered at the back of the neck and at the waist. Trimmed with satin stitch embroidery in colored silk in a rose spray and oak leaf design. Last quarter of the 19th century. Russian work.
Inv. No. E/rt-8673. Acquired in 1941.
The Hermitage

434. Morning Dress
White lawn. With train. Bodice fastening in front, square decolletage and sleeves opening to a broad flounce. Broad frill around the skirt's hem. Trimmed in white work. Late 19th–early 20th century.
Inv. No. E/rt-9444. Acquired in 1941.
The Hermitage

435. Ball Dress (bodice and skirt)
Bluish green panne. Belted, with exaggerated overlap of the blouse in front; low-necked, and short-sleeved. The skirt has a train. Trimmed with lace and sequins. 1900s. The workshop of N. Lamanova, Moscow.
Inv. No. E/rt-9463 a, b. Acquired in 1941.
The Hermitage

436. Ball Dress
Ivory velvet. Bias cut, low-necked, with short balloon sleeves. Trimmed with net worked with gold sequins and embroidered with imitation pearls, beadwork, and gold thread. 1890s. The workshop of A. T. Ivanova, St. Petersburg.
Inv. No. E/rt-12899. Acquired in 1941.

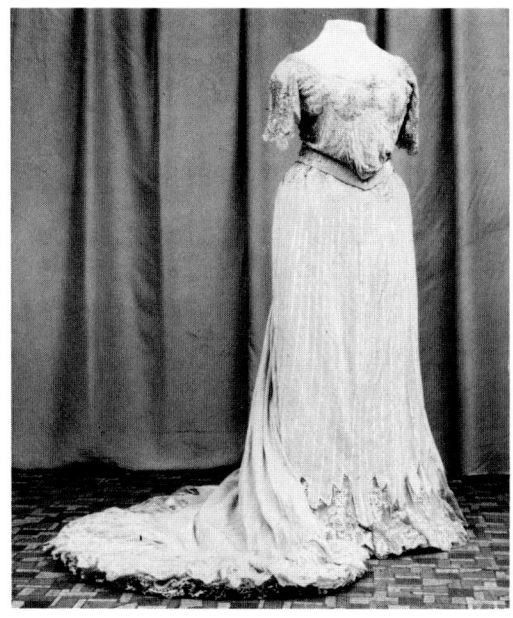

435

437. EVENING CLOAK Dark green velvet. With a standing collar; the back is slashed to show the train of the dress worn underneath. Trimmed with matching ostrich plumes and fringes of silk and beads.
Inv. No. E/rt-8581. Acquired in 1941.
The Hermitage

438. Dress (bodice and skirt)
White satin and silk tulle. Low-necked with elbow-length kimono sleeves. Overskirt is embroidered in white silk. 1910s. The workshop of N. Lamanova, Moscow.
Inv. No. E/rt-18057. Acquired in 1971.

439. BOA White ostrich plumes and down. Early 20th century.
Inv. No. E/rt-10299. Acquired in 1941.
The Hermitage

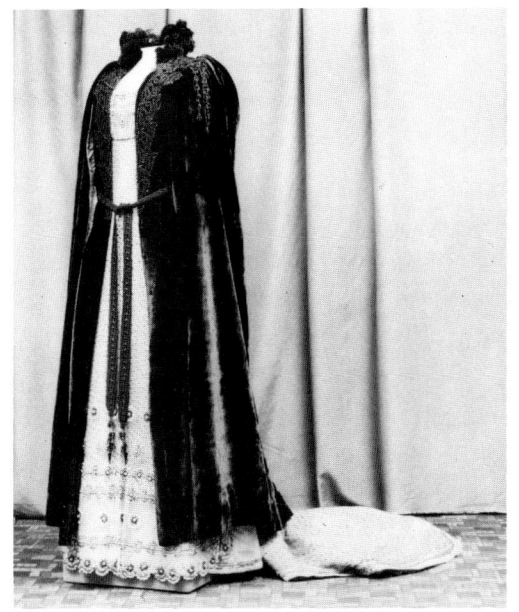 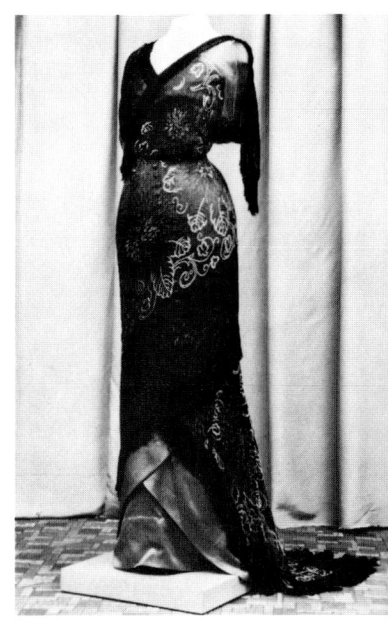

436, 437   440

440. **Dress** (bodice and skirt)
Black chiffon and green satin. V-necked decolletage and kimono sleeves. Narrow asymmetrically draped skirt flowing into the train. Trimmed with black fringe and embroidery worked in gold thread and silk. 1913–1914. The workshop of N. Lamanova, Moscow.
Inv. No. E/rt-18063 a, b. Acquired in 1972.
The Hermitage

441. **Dress**
Ivory panne and tulle. Low-necked, sleeveless, with straight narrow skirt slit in front at hem with an overskirt. Trimmed with artificial flowers, hand-crocheted, metallic thread, and embroidered in bugle beads. 1913. The firm of Paul Poiret, Paris.
Inv. No. E/rt-18054. Acquired in 1971.

105

442. EVENING CAPE Pink tulle. Adorned with beadwork and trimmed with marabou along the edges. Early 20th century.
Inv. No. E/rt-8221. Acquired in 1941.
The Hermitage

Fancy Dress in the Style of a Russian Man's Holiday Dress of the 17th Century
Rubakha, trousers, and hat executed by the firm "Brothers Leifert," St. Petersburg.
443. CAFTAN Silver brocade. With a peaked collar. Trimmed with velvet, gold galloon, beads, and strips of silk cord finished with spun gold tassels.
Inv. No. E/rt-13399. Acquired in 1941.
444. RUBAKHA White corded silk. With standing collar. Trimmed with gold cord and colored glass.
Inv. No. E/rt-13396. Acquired in 1941.
445. LONG TROUSERS Green plush. Trimmed with stripes of silver brocade worked with imitation pearls and glass.
Inv. No. E/rt-13391. Acquired in 1941.
446. HAT White satin. Silver brocade flap embroidered with imitation pearls and glass.
Inv. No. E/rt-13419. Acquired in 1941.
447. GLOVES (pair) Cuffs of yellow suede embroidered with gold thread and trimmed with fringe.
Inv. No. E/rt-13779 a, b. Acquired in 1941.
448. HIGH BOOTS (pair) Multicolored box calf leather. Low-heeled, decorated with outline pattern embroidery worked with colored threads. Late 19th century.
Inv. No. E/rt-13427 a, b. Acquired in 1941.
The Hermitage

Fancy Dress in the Style of a Russian Woman's Holiday Dress of the 17th Century
449. LETNIK (outer garment) Open at the front, with wide sleeves of purple satin, embroidered with gold and silver thread. Sleeves are trimmed with gold embroidery and fringe.
Inv. No. E/rt-13434. Acquired in 1941.
450. DRESS White silk with sleeves of white gauze. Opening in front, with a necklace (noticeably modernized). Trimmed with silver

brocade and embroidered with silk cord, threads, spun gold, mother-of-pearl, and spangles.
Inv. No. E/rt-13742. Acquired in 1941.
451. HAT Brocade embroidered with gold and silver threads. Round. Late 19th century.
Inv. No. E/rt-13422. Acquired in 1941.
The Hermitage

452. Shawl
Double-faced woven wool, with a sewn border. A floral pattern of lilac sprays. Double-headed eagle with St. George and the letters N. M. (Nadezhda Merlina) are woven in the right-hand corner. Work of serf craftsmen. First half of the 19th century. Size: 139 x 137 cm.
Inv. No. 55753 D-46.
Historical Museum

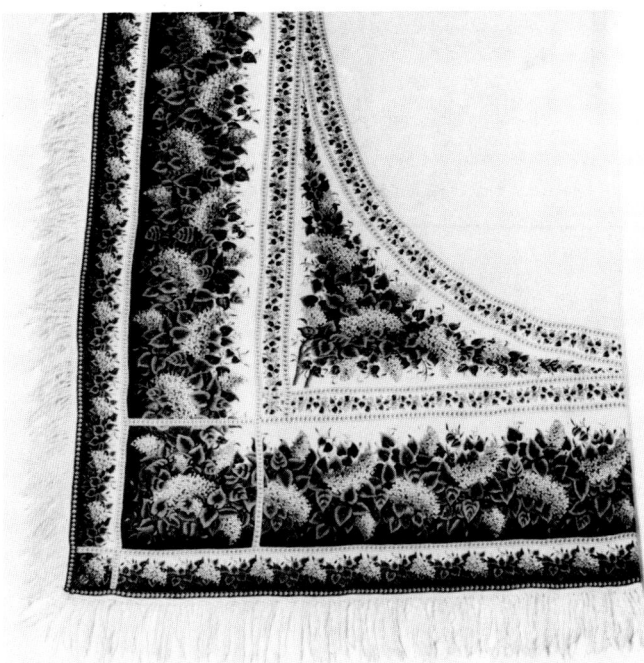

452

453. **Ornamental Band** (fragment of a shawl)
Double-faced woven wool with floral pattern on white background. Work of serf craftsmen. First quarter of the 19th century. Size: 276 x 10 cm.
Inv. No. 97108 D-1105. Acquired in 1960.
Historical Museum

454. **Ornamental Band** (fragment of a shawl)
Double-faced woven wool with floral pattern. Work of serf craftsmen. First half of the 19th century.
Inv. No. 55753 D-51. Acquired in 1929.
Historical Museum

455. **Hat**
Crimson straw decorated with beadwork. 1910s.
Inv. No. E/rt-6042. Acquired in 1941.
The Hermitage

456. **Hat**
Black straw. Wide-brimmed. Trimmed with ostrich plumes and a rose made of silver brocade. Early 20th century. Russian work.
Inv. No. E/rt-6052.
The Hermitage

457. **Gloves**
White kid with pierced gauntlet. Second half of the 19th century.
Inv. No. E/rt-12317 a, b. Acquired in 1941.
The Hermitage

458. **Gloves**
Black kid. Second half of the 19th century.
Inv. No. E/rt-6936 a, b. Acquired in 1941.
The Hermitage

459. **Stockings** (pair)
Black silk with multicolored flowers. Second half of the 19th century.

Inv. No. E/rt-2567 a, b. Acquired in 1941.
The Hermitage

460. Stockings (pair)
Mauve silk with black lace insets. Second half of the 19th century.
Inv. No. E/rt-2583 a, b. Acquired in 1941.
The Hermitage

461. Stockings (pair)
Red silk. Second half of the 19th century.
Inv. No. E/rt-2591 a, b. Acquired in 1941.
The Hermitage

462. Stockings (pair)
Golden yellow silk with white embroidery. Second half of the 19th century.
Inv. No. E/rt-2601 a, b. Acquired in 1941.
The Hermitage

463. Stockings (pair)
Peach silk with drawnwork and embroidered with forget-me-nots. Second half of the 19th century.
Inv. No. E/rt-2588 a, b. Acquired in 1941.
The Hermitage

464. Cape
Black woven lace. With hood and long ends. Second half of the 19th century. Russian work. Size: 68 x 223 cm.
Inv. No. E/rt-17564. Acquired in 1969.
The Hermitage

465. Cape
Black tulle embroidered with colored silk. 1820–1830s. Russia. Size: 47 x 132 cm.
Inv. No. E/rt-13983. Acquired in 1941.
The Hermitage

466. Mantlet
White tulle with satin stitch embroidery and lawn appliqué on tulle. 1840s. Russian work. Size: 105 x 234 cm.
Inv. No. E/rt-16905. Acquired in 1962.
The Hermitage

467. Cape
White tulle with chain stitch embroidery and lawn appliqué. Round. 1840–1850s. Russian work. Size: 28 x 78 cm.
Inv. No. E/rt-7587. Acquired in 1941.
The Hermitage

468. Scarf
Lace, knitted of black silk threads. Second half of the 19th century. Balakhna (?).
Inv. No. E/rt-17693. Acquired in 1970.
The Hermitage

469. Cape
Lace, cream silk thread. Late 19th century. St. Petersburg, village of Zakhozhye. Size: 110 x 250 cm.
Inv. No. E/rt-17218. Acquired in 1965.
The Hermitage

470. Handkerchief
White lawn decorated with white work and bordered with lace. First half of the 19th century. Size: 61 x 61 cm.
Inv. No. E/rt-8112. Acquired in 1941.
The Hermitage

471. Handkerchief
White lawn decorated with white work. 1850–1860s. Russia. Size: 45 x 45 cm.
Inv. No. E/rt-10242. Acquired in 1950.
The Hermitage

472. Garters (for stockings)
White satin with chain stitch embroidery worked in colored silk. Early 18th century. Russia. Size: 5.5 x 32.7 cm.

Inv. No. E/rt-8833 a, b. Acquired in 1941.
The Hermitage

473. Bag
White satin embroidered with colored silk and metallic thread worked in satin stitch. The design is of a park landscape.
Inv. No. E/rt-17827.
The Hermitage

474. Bag (pouch)
Yellow silk embroidered with metallic and silk threads worked in chain stitch. The design represents a vase with flowers and birds. Late 18th century. Russia. Size: 21.5 x 15.6 cm.
Inv. No. E/rt-5205. Acquired in 1941.
The Hermitage

475. Bag (pouch)
Pink silk embroidered with gold thread. Round. Late 18th-early 19th century. Russia. Size: 12.3 x 14 cm.
Inv. No. E/rt-4690. Acquired in 1941.
The Hermitage

476. Bag
Brown silk decorated with beadwork. Design of hunting scenes and landscape. The first third of the 19th century. Russia. Size: 27.5 x 19 cm.
Inv. No. E/rt-4864. Acquired in 1941.
The Hermitage

477. Wallet
White satin embroidered with silk and gold thread and tiny spangles. Lined with pink silk; with pink silk ribbon. 1798. Russia.
Inv. No. 69986 v-506. Acquired in 1930.
Historical Museum

478. Wallet
White satin embroidered with colored silk. Lined with white silk; with mauve silk ribbon. Early 20th century. Russia.
Inv. No. 69987 V-508. Acquired in 1930.
Historical Museum

479. Fan
Silk lined with paper. Painted in water colors and embroidered with spangles. The frame is of mother-of-pearl, decorated with carving, gilt, and silver. Mid-18th century. Length: 28.5 cm.
Inv. No. E/rt-6558. Acquired in 1941.
The Hermitage

480. Fan
Silk. Painted in water colors and embroidered with spangles. The frame is of ivory, with chased design and gilt work. Second half of the 18th century. Russia. Length: 27.3 cm.
Inv. No. E/rt-6597. Acquired in 1941.
The Hermitage

481. Fan
Pale yellow horn sticks, pierced and inlaid with steel spangles. Held together by a red ribbon. First third of the 19th century. Length: 15.5 cm.
Inv. No. E/rt-6481. Acquired in 1941.
The Hermitage

482. Fan
Lacelike cast-iron sticks held together by a black silk ribbon. Work of Kaslinskiye craftsmen. 1830–1840s. Russia.
Inv. No. E/rt-6764. Acquired in 1941.
The Hermitage

483. Large Fan
Blue feathers and white down.
Inv. No. E/rt-6675.
The Hermitage

484. Fan
Dark tortoiseshell sticks held together by black silk ribbon. Early 20th century. Length: 23 cm.
Inv. No. E/rt-6493. Acquired in 1974.
The Hermitage

485. Fan
White tulle ornamented with chain stitch embroidery. The

sticks are of carved ivory. Late 19th-early 20th century. Length: 36 cm.
Inv. No. E/rt-17092. Acquired in 1964.
The Hermitage

486. **Fan**
Gauze painted in purple-toned water colors with floral design of pansies. The frame is made of mother-of-pearl, with chased and painted floral ornament. Late 19th century. Length: 35.2 cm.
Inv. No. E/rt-6454. Acquired in 1941.
The Hermitage

487. **Fan**
Black gauze embroidered with metallic spangles. The frame is made of dark tortoiseshell. Early 20th century. Length: 23 cm.
Inv. No. E/rt-18363. Acquired in 1974.
The Hermitage

Tortoiseshell Set
Consists of four items. 1860s or 70s.
488. COMB Tortoiseshell inlaid with gold and silver.
Inv. No. ERO-8923. Acquired in 1964.
489. NECKLACE Tortoiseshell. In the form of round medallions and oval pendants encrusted with gold and silver. The spacer rings are gold.
Inv. No. ERO-8924 ZV-1350. Acquired in 1964.
490. EARRINGS (pair) Tortoiseshell. Oval, with a bow, encrusted with gold and silver. Lock is gold.
Inv. Nos. ERO-8925 a, b. ZV-1351 a, b. Acquired in 1964.
491. FAN Tortoiseshell. With a gold monogram "A.S." The pivot is gold.
Inv. Nos. ERO-8926 ZV-1352. Acquired in 1964.
The Hermitage

492. **Earrings** (pair)
Silver gilt set with turquoise and pearls. 1860s.
Inv. No. EPO-2280 a, b. SV-3216. Acquired in 1941.
The Hermitage

493. **Earrings**
Silver filigree. With three-piece spherical fringed pendant. Second half of the 19th century.
Inv. No. ERO-2255 a, b. SV-3438. Acquired in 1941.
The Hermitage

494. **Earrings**
Silver gilt set with garnets and pearls. 1860s.
Inv. No. ERO-2260 SV-214, 215. Acquired in 1941.
The Hermitage

495. **Earrings** (pair)
Silver gilt with river pearls. 18th century. Russian work.
Inv. No. ERO-8839 a, b SV-4206.
The Hermitage

496. **Earrings** (pair)
Amber set in chased gold. Second half of the 19th century.
Inv. No. ERO-6118, a, b ZV-493. Acquired in 1941.
The Hermitage

497. **Brooch**
Amber rectangle set in gold. Second half of the 19th century.
Inv. No. ERO-6117 ZV-492. Acquired in 1941.
The Hermitage

498. **Brooch**
Silver gilt set with garnets and pearls. 1860s.
Inv. No. ERO-2265 SV-223. Acquired in 1941.
The Hermitage

499. **Brooch**
Silver gilt set with turquoise and pearls. 1860s.
Inv. No. ERO-2283 SV-2966. Acquired in 1941.
The Hermitage

500. **Necklace**
Silver filigree with pendants suspended on a fine chain. Bow-shaped. Second half of the 19th century.
Inv. No. ERO-2312 SB-496. Acquired in 1941.
The Hermitage

501. **Necklace**
Silver gilt decorated with a filigree ornament representing a bunch of flowers, with pendants, attached by chain; inlaid with a floral and leaf motif. Second half of the 19th century.
Inv. No. ERO-2310 SB-494. Acquired in 1941.
The Hermitage

502. **Bracelet**
Blued steel with plated bronze and steel "diamonds." First half of the 19th century. Tula.
Inv. No. E/rm-4097. Acquired in 1941.
The Hermitage

503. **Bracelets** (pair)
Braided wire with buckles and locks of cast iron. Worn over sleeves. 1830–1840s. The Urals, village of Kasli.
Inv. Nos. E/rm-4899, 4900. Acquired in 1941.
The Hermitage

504. **Bracelet**
Silver set with garnets, pearls, and an almandine in the center. 1860s.
Inv. No. ERO-6115 ZV-456. Acquired in 1941.
The Hermitage

505. **Bracelet**
Multicolored agate. Four sections shaped like buckles with two pendants of agate beads. 19th century. Russia.
Inv. No. E/rkm-887. Acquired in 1941.
The Hermitage

506. **Necklace**
Cast iron. Sections in the shape of rosettes and palmettes. 1830–1840s. The Urals, village of Kasli.
Inv. No. E/rt-808. Acquired in 1941.
The Hermitage

507. **Beads**
Malachite. First half of the 19th century. Russia.
Inv. No. E/rtkp-333. Acquired in 1941.
The Hermitage

508. Beads
Cut rock crystal. 19th century. Russia.
Inv. No. E/ram-573. Acquired in 1941.
The Hermitage

509. Belt
Braided wire with cast-iron buckle. 1830s. The Urals, village of Kasli.
Inv. No. E/rm-4898. Acquired in 1941.
The Hermitage

510. Comb
Tortoiseshell. 1830s.
Inv. No. E/rt-16805. Acquired in 1960.
The Hermitage

511. Two Hairpins
Tortoiseshell. Second half of the 19th century.
Inv. Nos. E/rr-580, 581. Acquired in 1941.
The Hermitage

512. Nosegay Holder
Decorated with enamel and set with turquoises and garnets. Mid-19th century.
Inv. No. E/rt-861. Acquired in 1941.
The Hermitage

513. Nosegay Holder
Tortoiseshell decorated with gold. Mid-19th century.
Inv. No. E/rt-363. Acquired in 1941.
The Hermitage